Oh's

오지은의 메디컬 영어회화

.General Hospital

part.2

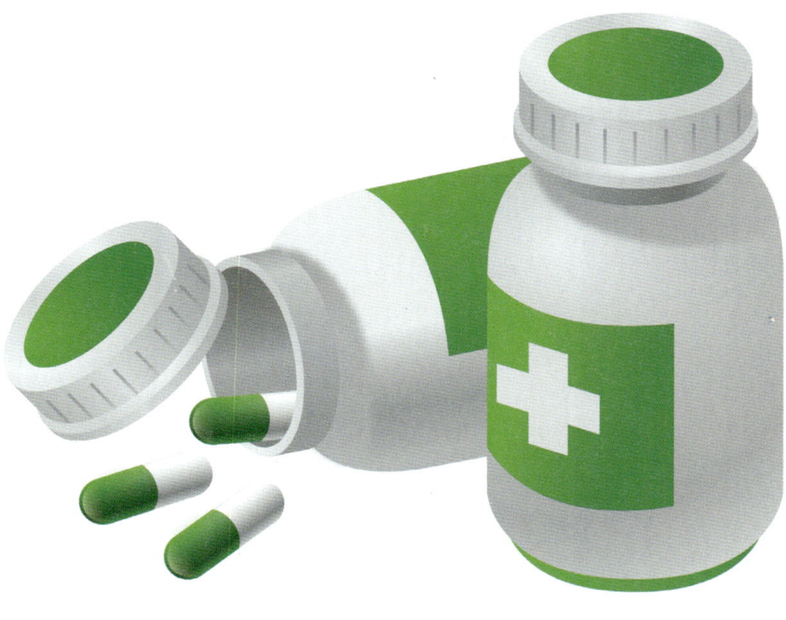

청구문화사

오지은의 메디컬 영어회화 part 2

2011년 6월 15일 초판인쇄
2011년 6월 25일 초판발행

지은이 / 오지은
펴낸이 / 이상태
펴낸곳 / 청구문화사
120-831 서울특별시 서대문구 연희1동 436-1
전 화 / 02) 332-0541(代)
팩 스 / 02) 337-9577
등 록 / 1990년 11월 2일 제9-247호

ISBN 978-89-5616-447-2 93510

정가 35,000원

The Story of 오지은의 메디컬 영어회화. General Hospital

오지은의 메디컬 영어회화. General Hospital은 2009년 4월부터 시작하여 2011년 1월 7일에 완성한 저의 첫 번째 메디컬 영어회화책인 종합병원 편입니다.

이 책은 두 가지의 숙제를 풀고 싶은 마음에서 집필하였습니다. 첫 번째 숙제는, 의료 통역이란 난제의 답을 찾는 실마리가 되어 의료관광이라는 현장에서 선구자의 역할을 하시는 의료 통역사/의료통역 코디네이터 분들에게 영어권 환자분들의 의료 및 생활 문화와 현지의 살아있는 영어를 알려드리고 싶었습니다. "영어권 환자들은 어디에서 왔는가?" 란 질문에 대한 답을 아실 때 의료통역은 한결 더 수월해지실 것이라 생각됩니다. 두 번째 숙제는 해외에 특히 미국으로 진출하시려는 의료종사자분 들의 "우리는 어디로 가는가?"에 대한 답을 드리고 싶었습니다. 저는 미국 대학에서 세포병리학을 전공했고 세포병리사로 미국의 병리 연구 산업기관과 지역병원에서 근무를 하였습니다. 아는 만큼 보인다는 격언이 있듯이 십여 년이 넘는 제 미국생활의 경험을 미국의 의료 시장으로 진출을 준비하시고 계시는 분들께 알려드리고 싶었습니다. 미국에 도착 후 가장 먼저 만들어야 하는 Social Security Card를 Chapter 1에 실은 이유도 여기에 있습니다. 언어는 문화입니다.

그리고 세 번째의 숙제를 추가하자면 아직 재학중인 보건계열 학생 여러분들이 졸업 전에 이 책을 공부하고 졸업 후 내딛는 사회의 첫 발에 도움이 되었으면 하는 바람입니다. "영어는 권력이다" 라는 항간에 회자되는 말에 저는 영어는 "많은 문을 열어 줄 수 있는 열쇠이다"를 첨가하고 싶습니다.

끝으로 감사의 말을 전하고 싶습니다. 현재 의료 현장에 근무하시며 각자의 꿈을 이루기 위해 향학열을 불태우시는 소중한 오지은의 메디컬 영어회화 1기생인, 김

수민, 최현경, 허선희, 장수경간호사님과 특히 제게 한국의료문화에 대해 많은 조언을 주는 나의 동지인 순천향대학병원의 송선주 간호사님께 큰 감사를 드립니다. 또한 이비인후과 박상철 의사선생님, 조현재 치과 의사선생님, 조욱 심장내과 의사선생님, 수원 아주 대학교병원의 약사님, 서울아산병원의 김주연 간호사님, 박소영 의료통역사님, 최영주 아로마테라피 연구소장님 외에 제 강의를 수강하신 모든 분들의 소중한 자문으로 이 책이 세상 밖에 나올 수 있었습니다. 현장의 소리를 담은 책이 되고 싶은 제 꿈을 그 분들이 가능하게 해 주셨습니다. 그리고 가장 핵심 과제였던 이 책이 지향하는 방향을 설정하는데 사려 깊은 조언을 주신 정동혁 병원경영 컨설턴트님께 깊은 감사와 고마움을 전합니다.

메디컬 외국어 회화를 처음으로 한국대학교에 개설하신 김천대학교의 의료경영학과 박지원 학과장님과 청구문화사 이상태 사장님을 비롯한 직원들의 노고에 깊이 감사를 드립니다.

이 책의 제목, 표지 디자인 및 다양한 콘텐츠를 이용하실 수 있는 www.ohgieun.com 홈페이지는 B&M Company의 작품입니다. 그들은 천재입니다. 그들에게 무한한 감사의 마음을 전합니다.

Introduction

Part 2는 외국인 환자분들과 의사와의 진료상담을 소개하였습니다. 진료실에서 그들의 증상과 통증에 관한 다양한 질문과 그에 상응하는 답변 및 진단 후 내려지는 복약지시에 관한 소개로 구성되어 있습니다.

네 번째 장인 증상에서는 외국인 환자분들이 병원을 내원하여 진료실에서 그들의 증상을 설명하는 상황을 소개하였습니다. 증상에 관한 주요어휘, 주요구문, 및 각 상황에 맞는 대화로 구성하였습니다.

다섯 번째 장은 통증입니다. 통증관련 주요어휘와 통증의 기간 및 통증의 완화, 악화의 원인에 관한 상황을 상세히 분류하여 외국인 환자의 문진에 대비하실 수 있도록 여러 표현들을 준비하였습니다. 또한 통증에 관련된 독해구문과 통증척도표의 역사도 간략히 소개하였습니다.

여섯 번째 장은 복약지시에 관한 것입니다. 증상과 통증에 근거한 문진 후 내려지는 복약지시에 관한 내용을 주요어휘, 주요구문, 대화구문, 미국 처방전의 견본 및 비처방전 약의 설명서로 구성하였습니다.

Part 2의 증상, 통증 및 복약지시관련 표현은 Part 3의 진료 후 검사로 이어집니다. Part 3는 **Chapter 7: 혈액검사 및 소변검사**, **Chapter 8: 엑스레이 검사**와 **Chapter 9: 활력징후**로 구성하였습니다. **Part 3**에서 뵙겠습니다.

Special Thanks

Without the Karls, I couldn't finish my first book.

I really appreciate all of your help and support.

Synghoon Karl

Ji-Won Karl

Min-Kyu Karl

Love,

From the bottom of my heart

Part 2

Contents

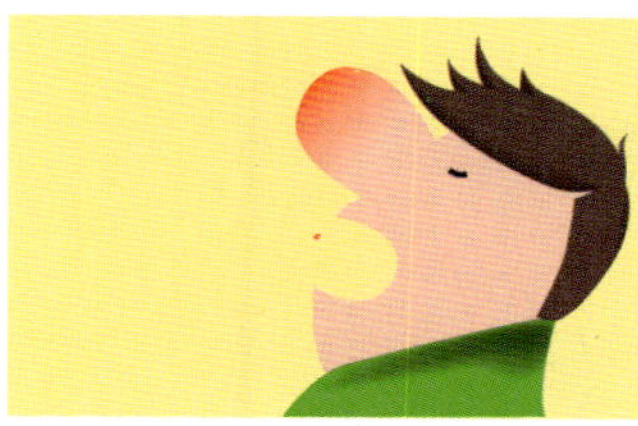

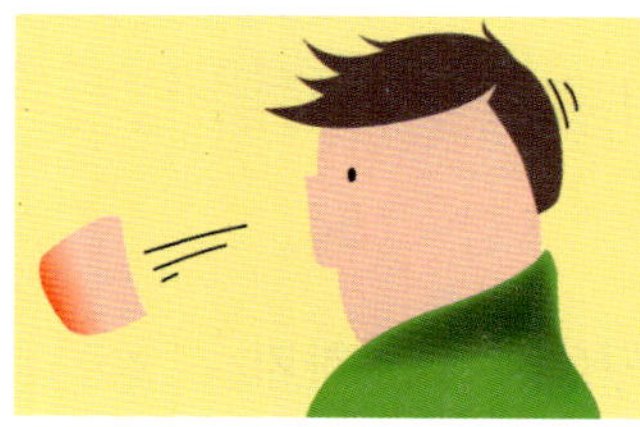

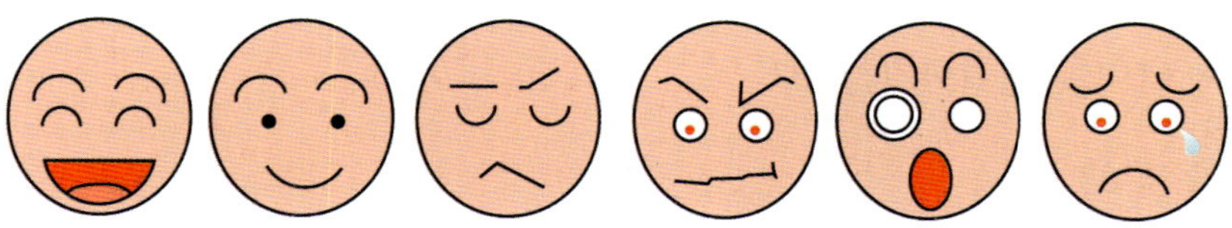

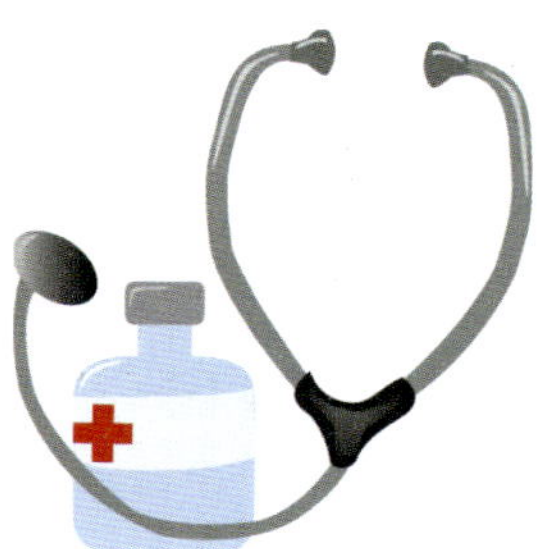

Contents

Chapter 4. Symptoms

1. Types of Symptoms, 증상의 종류

2. A List of Key Expression for Symptoms: 증상표현 주요구문 모음

3. Story of My Symptoms, 나의 증상 이야기

4. Frequently Asked Questions for My Symptoms, 증상에 관해 자주하는 질문

5. Describing My Symptoms, 나의 증상 설명하기

Contents

5. Timing of Pain, 통증발생 시간

Contents

6. Intensity of Pain, 통증의 강도

7. Pain Scale from 0-10, 통증척도표 0-1 0

10. Alleviation & Aggravation of Pain, 통증의 완화 및 **악화**

2. Prescription, 처방전

Contents

5. FAQ at the pharmacy, 약국에서 자주하는 질문 모음

6. Over-the-Counter Medication, 비처방전 약

7. 정답 및 해석

Chapter 4
Symptoms
증상

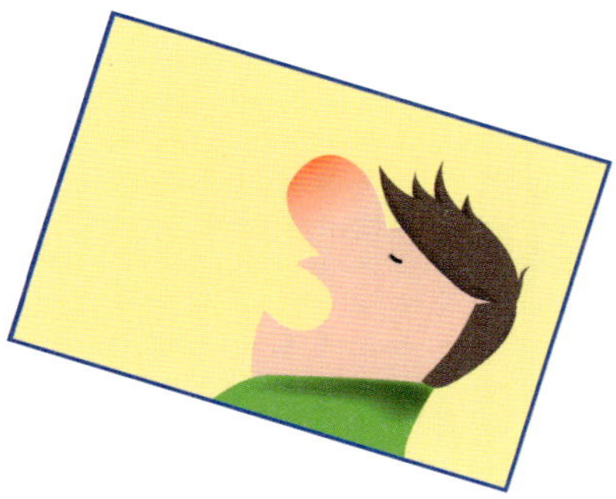

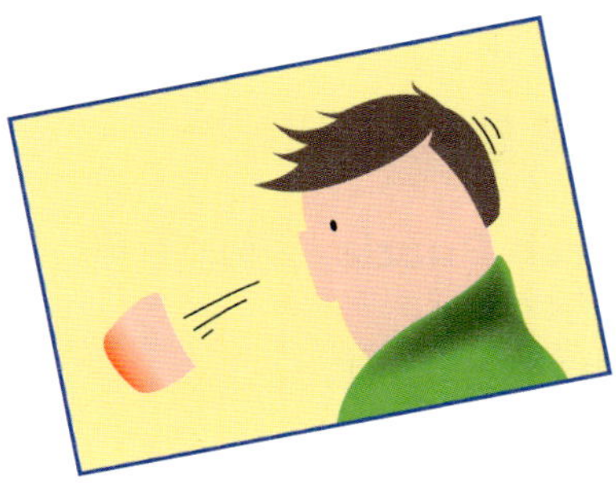

1. Types of Symptoms 증상의 종류

- **Key Words, 주요어휘**

  A. 피로
  B. 소화기 질환
     - Quiz: 내 단어장 점검하기
  C. 호흡기 질환
  D. 감기 및 독감
     - Quiz: 내 단어장 점검하기
  E. 관절 질환
  F. 피부 질환
     - Quiz: 내 단어장 점검하기
  G. 빈혈
  H. 안 질환
     - Quiz: 내 단어장 점검하기
  I. 기타
     - Quiz: 내 단어장 점검하기

- **Drill: Word Search Puzzle, 연습문제: 어휘퍼즐**

  J. 유아 관련 질환 증상
     - Quiz: 내 단어장 점검하기
     - Drill: Word Search Puzzle, 연습문제: 어휘퍼즐

- **Word Review, 어휘복습**

Key Words

A. 피로

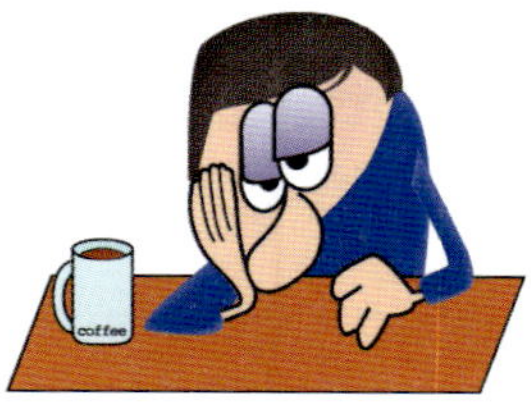

Exhausted: 지친, 힘이 없는

Sluggish: 나른한

Lethargy: 매우 지친, 탈수로 늘어진

Fatigue, Tiredness: 피곤함

B. 소화기 질환

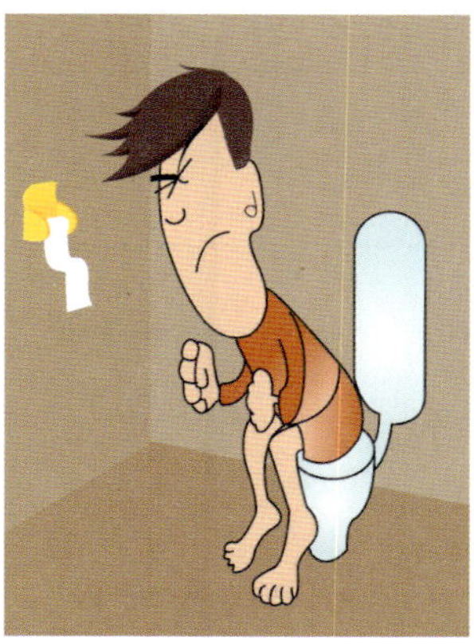

Enema: 관장

Nauseous (Queasy): 메스꺼운

Bowel movement(s): 대변을 보는 것

Constipation (Irregularity): 변비

Heartburn: 속 쓰림

Vomiting (Puke, Throwing up): 구토

Diarrhea (Having the runs): 설사

Lose one's appetite: 식욕이 없다

Weight loss: 체중감소

Dehydration: 탈수

Bloated: 복부팽만감이 있는

QUIZ: 내 단어장 점검하기 !!

아래 단어 및 구문을 읽고 알맞은 증상의 이름을 적어보세요.

Vomiting: ....

Exhausted: ....

Bowel movement(s): ....

Sluggish: ....

Queasy: ....

Lethargy: ....

Fatigue, Tiredness: ....

Diarrhea: ....

Puke: ....

Throwing up: ....

Enema: ....

Nauseous: ....

Constipation: ....

Heartburn: ....

Lose one's appetite: ....

Weight loss: ....

Irregularity: ....

Dehydration: ....

Bloated: ....

Having the runs: ....

C. 호흡기 질환

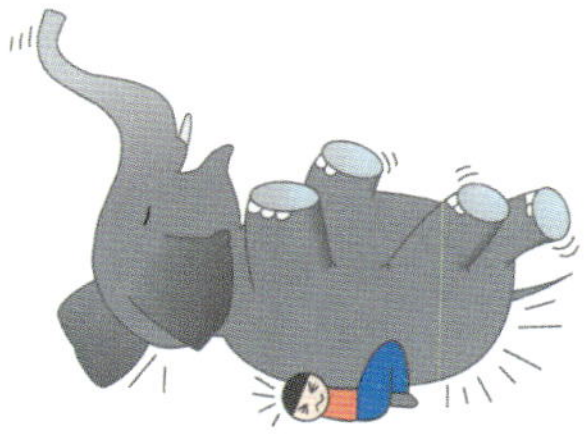

Shortness of breath (Rapid breathing): 숨이 찬

Wheeze: 숨을 쌕쌕 거리다

Asthma: 천식

D. 감기 및 독감

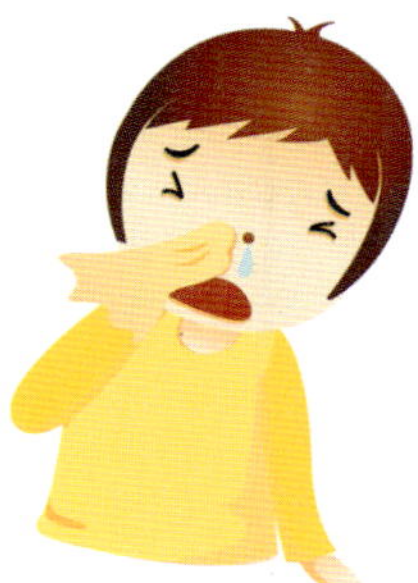

Cough: 기침

Cold sweat: 식은땀

Stuffy nose (Congestion): 코가 막힘

Sore throat: 인후염

Scratchy sensation in the back of one's throat:
목안이 쓰리고 까끌까끌 거리는

Chills: 오한

Fever: 발열

Feverish: 열이 나는

Drowsy: 졸리운

Sweat, Perspiration: 땀, 발한

Hoarse: 목소리가 쉰

Body aches: 몸살

A cold: 감기

Seasonal flu: 계절성 독감

QUIZ: 내 단어장 점검하기 !!

아래 단어 및 구문을 읽고 알맞은 증상의 이름을 적어보세요.

Shortness of breath: ....

Rapid breathing: ....

Wheeze: ....

Asthma: ....

Cough: ....

Cold sweat: ....

Stuffy nose: ....

Congestion: ....

Sore throat: ....

Chills: ....

Fever: ....

Feverish: ....

Drowsy: ....

Sweat: ....

Perspiration: ....

Hoarse: ....

Body aches: ....

A cold: ....

Seasonal flu: ....

Scratchy sensation in the back of one's throat: ....

....

E. 관절 질환

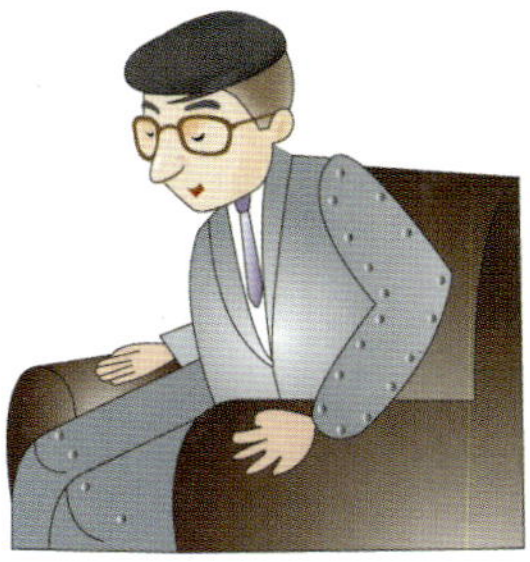

Stiff: 뻣뻣한

Morning stiffness: 아침에 몸이 뻣뻣한

Joint stiffness: 관절이 뻣뻣한

F. 피부 질환

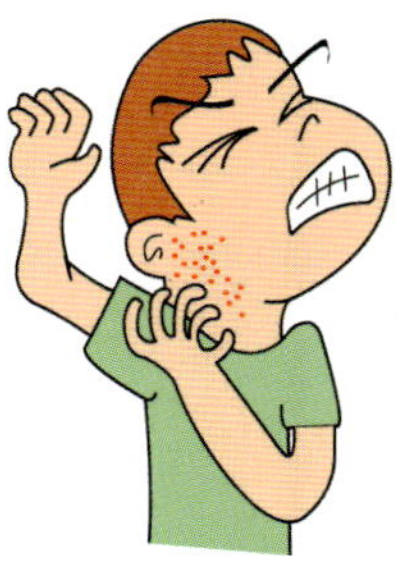

Rash: 발진

Heat rash: 땀띠

Inflamed area: 염증부위

Scarred: 흉터가 있는

Swollen/Edema: 부어 있는/부종

Dry and cracked skin: 건조하고 갈라진 피부

Irritated skin: 염증이 생긴 피부

Blister/Bulla: 수포

Discharge: 분비물

Pus: 고름, 농포

Burning sensation: 따끔따끔한

Numb: 감각이 무딘

Hives: 두드러기

QUIZ: 내 단어장 점검하기 !!

아래 단어 및 구문을 읽고 알맞은 증상의 이름을 적어보세요.

Stiff: ....

Irritated skin: ....

Morning stiffness: ....

Pus: ....

Dry and cracked skin: ....

Rash: ....

Blister: ....

Heat rash: ....

Inflamed area: ....

Scarred: ....

Hives: ....

Swollen: ....

Bulla: ....

Discharge: ....

Joint stiffness: ....

Burning sensation: ....

Edema: ....

Numb: ....

G. 빈혈

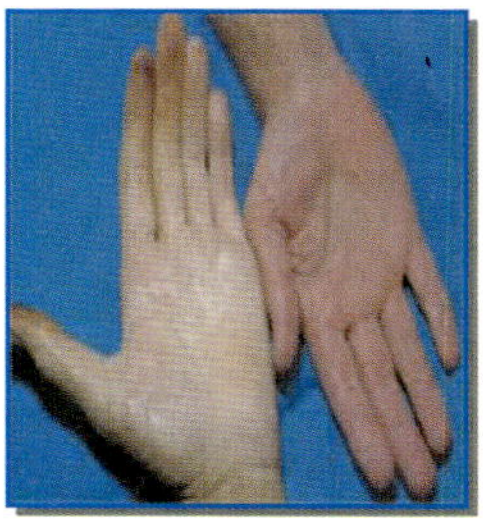

Anemia: 빈혈

Paleness (Pallor): 창백함

Pallor of the hand in anemia patient on the left and the physician's hand on the right.

H. 안 질환

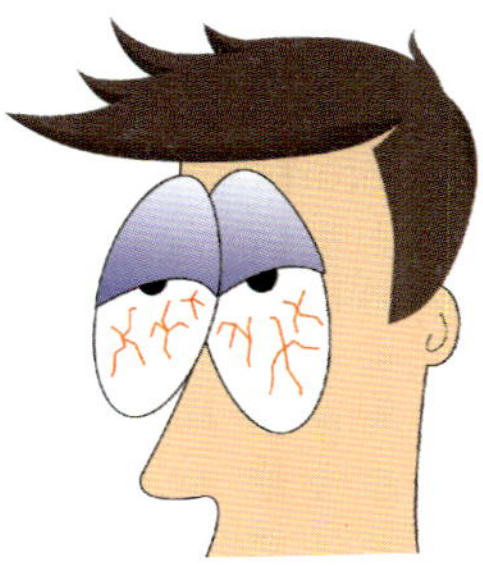

Pinky eyes/Conjunctivitis: 결막염

Itching eyes (Itchy eyes): 눈이 가려움

Yellow or green discharge from the eyes: 눈곱

Double vision: 복시, 사물이 두 개로 보이는

Blurred vision: 또렷이 보이지 않는

Hazy vision: 흐리고 뿌옇게 보이는

Dry eyes: 안구 건조증

Twitching eyelid: 눈꺼풀이 떨림

Bloodshot eyes: 충혈된 눈

Watering eyes (Teary): 눈물이 많이 나는 눈

Black eye: 멍든 눈

Stye: 다래끼

QUIZ: 내 단어장 점검하기 !!

아래 단어 및 구문을 읽고 알맞은 증상의 이름을 적어보세요.

Paleness: ....

Blurred vision: ....

Conjunctivitis: ....

Itching eyes: ....

Stye: ....

Twitching eyelid: ....

Double vision: ....

Pallor: ....

Dry eyes: ....

Anemia: ....

Pinky eyes: ....

Bloodshot eyes: ....

Itchy eyes: ....

Black eye: ....

Watering eyes: ....

Hazy vision: ....

Teary: ....

Yellow or green discharge from the eyes: ....

....

I. 기타

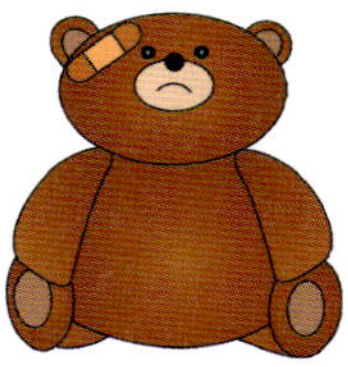

Heart pounding/Palpitation: 가슴이 두근거림/심계항진

Cyanosis: 청색증

Ringing in the ears/Tinnitus: 귀 울림/이명

Night sweats: 야간발한작용

Sleeplessness/Insomnia: 불면증

Dizziness (Lightheadedness, Dizzy spells): 현기증, 어질어질한

Faintness (Pass out): 실신

Burning sensation: 속 쓰림

Osmidrosis: 액취증

Hyperhidrosis: 다한증

Cluster headaches: 군집성 두통

Migraine headache (Migraine): 편두통

Heat stroke: 열사병

Bruise: 멍, 타박상

Nose bleed: 코피

Dry mouth: 구강건조증

Muscle spasm: 근육경련

Night sweats/Sleep Hyperhidrosis: 수면 중 과다하게 땀을 흘림

QUIZ: 내 단어장 점검하기 !!

아래 단어 및 구문을 읽고 알맞은 증상의 이름을 적어보세요.

Night sweats: ....

Palpitation: ....

Ringing in the ears: ....

Faintness: ....

Lightheadedness: ....

Dizzy spells: ....

Osmidrosis: ....

Insomnia: ....

Burning sensation: ....

Heart pounding: ....

Sleeplessness: ....

Cyanosis: ....

Dizziness: ....

Tinnitus: ....

Migraine: ....

Pass out: ....

Hyperhidrosis: ....

Cluster headaches: ....

Sleep Hyperhidrosis: ....

Heat stroke: ....

Bruise: ....

Migraine headache: ....

Nose bleed: ....

Dry mouth: ....

Muscle spasm: ....

Night sweats: ....

Chapter 4

Drill: 아래의 단어를 Word Search Puzzle에서 찾아보세요.

C	Q	N	C	H	I	L	L	S	Q	N	M	L	U	Q	U	P
Y	O	Q	U	E	A	S	Y	S	R	R	O	E	S	X	F	I
A	G	L	B	A	D	F	M	H	E	A	R	T	B	U	R	N
N	Q	Q	D	T	E	I	R	Q	D	W	N	H	A	P	G	K
O	Y	N	P		R	O	Z	B	I	K	I	A	A	S	B	Y
S	B	C	I	R	S	I	W	Z	X	U	N	R	W	E	S	
I	M	B	I	A	S	W	H	N	Y	M	G	G	T	A	E	E
S	B	H	J	S	I	K	E	P	Y			Y	O	S	F	Y
B	Q	A	C	H	L	H	E	A	T		S	T	R	O	K	E
G	N	T	B	J	I	Q	Z	L	T	A	T	P	L	N	P	S
H	G	L	W	V	Y	P	E	L	L	J	I	F	E	A	Y	N
W	T	K	E	N	J	W	P	O	K	E	F	R	Q	L	N	L
D	A	S	X	I	J	X	V	R	K	A	F	W	I		L	A
N	W	S	T	S	Q	K	O	S	R	S	N	X	C	F	X	S
M	T	W	I	T	C	H	I	N	G		E	Y	E	L	I	D
K	N	C	Y	W	P	Q	E	O	F	O	S	J	G	U	S	B
X	O	J	X	Q	L	T	R	J	Q	K	S	Q	W	Y	H	J

매우 지친/탈수로 늘어진, 속 쓰림, 메스꺼운, 숨을 쌕쌕 거리다, 식은땀, 오한, 계절성 독감, 아침에 몸이 뻣뻣한, 땀띠, 두드러기, 창백함, 결막염, 눈꺼풀이 떨림, 현기증, 열사병, 청색증

J. 유아 관련 질환 증상

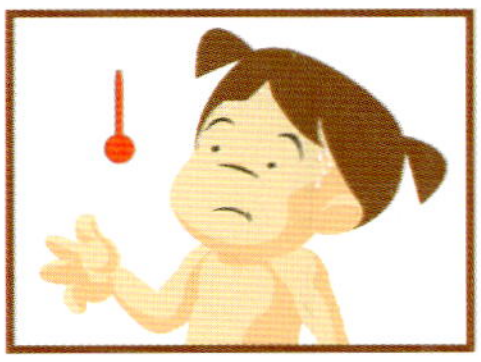

Fever: 열

Cold hands & feet: 손과 발이 차가운

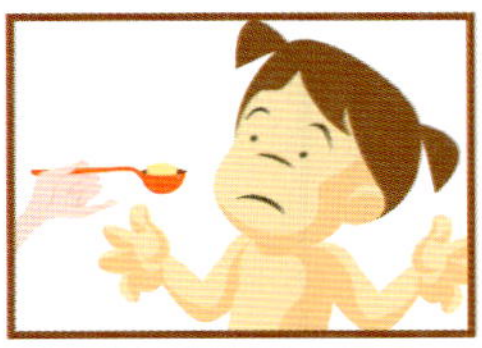

Refusing food: 음식을 거부하는

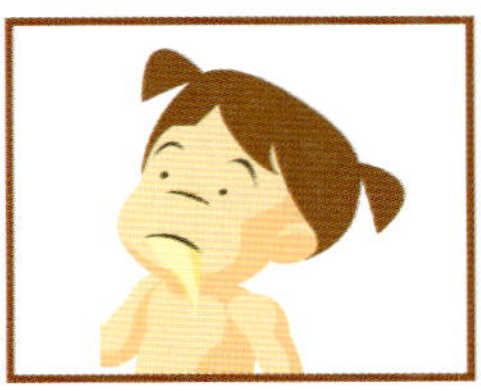

Vomiting: 구토

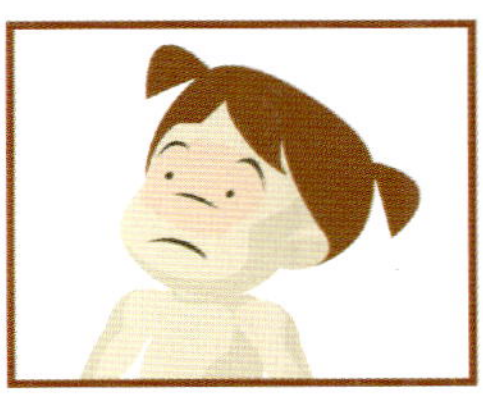

Pale skin: 피부가 창백한

Blotchy skin: 붉게 반점이 생긴

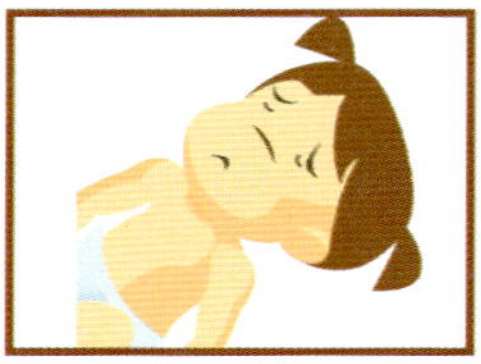

Floppy: 축 처진

Listless: 힘이 없는, 무기력한

Unresponsive: 반응하지 않는

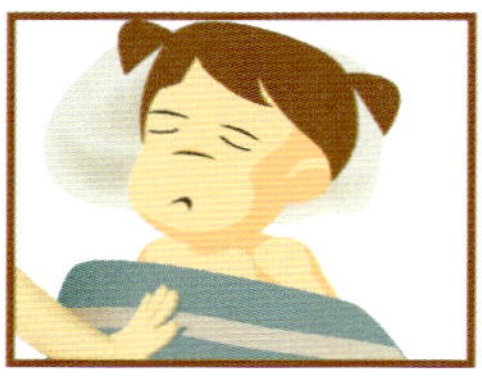

Drowsy: 졸린

Difficult to wake: 깨우기 힘든

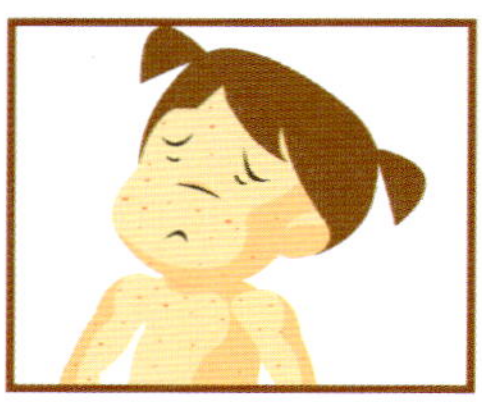

Spots: 반점

Rash: 발진

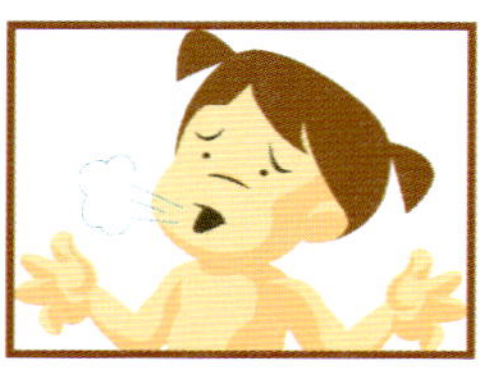

Rapid breathing: 숨이 가쁜

Grunting: 앓는 소리를 내는

QUIZ: 내 단어장 점검하기 !!

아래 단어 및 구문을 읽고 알맞은 증상의 이름을 적어보세요.

Fever: ....

Spots: ....

Refusing food: ....

Pale skin: ....

Blotchy skin: ....

Drowsy: ....

Cold hands & feet: ....

Floppy: ....

Unresponsive: ....

Rapid breathing: ....

Difficult to wake: ....

Vomiting: ....

Rash: ....

Listless: ....

Grunting: ....

Drill: 아래의 단어를 Word Search Puzzle에서 찾아보세요.

D	M	X	Y	L	F	J	N	K	B	U	M	R	P	H
Q	M	I	S	N	X	E	T	T	G	G	B	A	G	A
U	B	U	M	V	G	O	V	H	U	T	Q	P	C	Q
O	Q	L	V	A	T	X	I	E	N	R	Q	I	C	M
B	T	F	O	I	W	M	Y	F	R	M	E	D	J	E
G	R	U	N	T	I	N	G	A	E	L	X		G	D
P	U	W	P	M	C	G	S	Q	S	K	T	B	D	R
J	D	V	U	S	Q	H	P	R	P	A	G	R	U	I
P	B	Q	R	G	G	P	Y	N	O	M	O	E	R	S
Y	T	W	Q	Q	W	T	N		N	W	C	A	Q	N
E	D	L	I	S	T	L	E	S	S	P	O	T	S	G
E	C	G	R	F	A	R	S	Y	I	K	N	H	A	F
P	H	O	N	L	R	J	V	X	V	Q	I	I	Q	N
O	K	Q	S	H	V	P	J	S	E	W	B	N	C	A
N	J	C	G	E	V	O	M	I	T	I	N	G	T	N

구토, 붉게 반점이 생긴, 열, 앓는 소리를 내는, 반점, 발진, 힘이 없는/무기력한, 반응하지 않는, 졸린, 숨이 가쁜

Word Review: 위의 단어들을 복습하는 공간입니다.
정답은 Key Words를 참고하세요.

뜻: In English

지친, 힘이 없는:________________

나른한:________________

매우 지친, 탈수로 늘어진:________________

피곤함:________________

관장:________________

메스꺼운:________________

대변을 보는 것:________________

변비:________________

속 쓰림:________________

구토:________________

설사:________________

식욕이 없다:________________

체중감소:________________

탈수:________________

복부팽만감이 있는:________________

숨이 찬: ____________________

숨을 쌕쌕 거리다: ____________________

천식: ____________________

기침: ____________________

식은땀: ____________________

코가 막힘: ____________________

인후염: ____________________

목안이 쓰리고 까끌까끌 거리는: ____________________

오한: ____________________

발열: ____________________

졸리운: ____________________

열이 나는: ____________________

땀, 발한: ____________________

목소리가 쉰: ____________________

몸살: ____________________

감기: ____________________

계절성 독감: ____________________

뻣뻣한: ____________________

아침에 몸이 뻣뻣한: ____________________

관절이 뻣뻣한: ____________________

발진: ____________________

땀띠: ____________________

염증부위: ____________________

흉터가 있는: ____________________

부어 있는/부종: ____________________

건조하고 갈라진 피부: ____________________

염증이 생긴 피부: ____________________

수포: ____________________

분비물: ____________________

고름, 농포: ____________________

따끔따끔한: ____________________

감각이 무딘: ____________________

두드러기: ____________________

빈혈: ____________________

창백함: ____________________

결막염: ____________________

눈이 가려움: ____________________

눈곱: ____________________

복시, 사물이 두 개로 보이는: ____________________

또렷이 보이지 않는: ____________________

흐리고 뿌옇게 보이는: ____________________

안구 건조증: ____________________

눈꺼풀이 떨림: ____________________

충혈된 눈: ____________________

눈물이 많이 나는 눈: ____________________

멍든 눈: ____________________

다래끼: ____________________

가슴이 두근거림/심계항진: ____________________

청색증: ____________________

귀 울림/이명: ____________________

야간발한작용: ____________________

불면증: ____________________

현기증, 어질어질한: ____________________

실신: ____________________

속 쓰림: ____________________

액취증: ____________________

다한증: ____________________

군집성 두통: ____________________

편두통: ____________________

열사병:________________

멍, 타박상:________________

코피:________________

구강건조증:________________

근육경련:________________

수면 중 과다하게 땀을 흘림:________________

열:________________

손과 발이 차가운:________________

음식을 거부하는:________________

구토:________________

피부가 창백한:________________

붉게 반점이 생긴:________________

축 처진:________________

힘이 없는, 무기력한:________________

반응하지 않는:________________

졸린:________________

깨우기 힘든:________________

반점:________________

발진:________________

숨이 가쁜:________________

앓는 소리를 내는:________________

2. A List of Key Expressions for Symptoms: 증상표현 주요구문 모음

- **Key Expressions: "나는 ~한 증상이 있어요."**
    - I have + "Symptoms."
    - I Do/Be 동사 + "Symptoms"
    - My~ Do/Be 동사 + "Symptoms."
    - Right/Left/Both body part Do/Be 동사 + "Symptoms."
    - Words, 어휘
    - Drill, 연습문제

- **Key Expressions: " ~가 아프셔서 오셨나요?"/ " ~부위가 아프세요?"**
    - What~으로 시작하는 "~가 아프셔서 오셨나요?"
    - How~로 시작하는 "~가 아프셔서 오셨나요?"
    - Where/Which~로 시작하는 "~부위가 아프세요?"
    - Words, 어휘
    - Drill, 연습문제

Key Expressions: 나는 ~한 "증상"이 있어요.

I have + "Symptoms."

① I have the flu.

② I have a cold.

③ I have a runny nose.

④ I have chills.

⑤ I have a bad cough.

⑥ I have a rash.

⑦ I have a bad cut.

⑧ I have heartburn.

⑨ I have dry mouth.

⑩ I have indigestion.

⑪ I have had the runs for the past couple of days.

⑫ I often have a nose bleed in the morning.

⑬ I have muscle spasm.

⑭ I have been coughing up blood all day.

I have been bringing up blood all day.

⑮ I have difficulty in breathing.

Key Expressions: 나는 ~한 "증상"이 있어요.

I Do/Be 동사 + "Symptoms."

① **I ache** all over.

② **I sneeze** a lot.

③ **I feel** nauseous./**I feel** nauseated.

④ **I lost** all my appetite.

⑤ **I can't catch** my breath.

⑥ **I feel** dizzy all day.

⑦ **I'm** hoarse because of recent cold.

⑧ **I'm** tired all the time.

My ~ Do/Be 동사 + "Symptoms"

① **My eyes** itch.

② **My eyes** are teary.

③ **My eyes** are sensitive to light.

④ **My vision** is hazy.

⑤ My skin itches.

⑥ My lips are dry.

⑦ My throat is sore.

⑧ My stomach hurts.

⑨ My ears are clogged up.

⑩ My mouth feels dry and rough.

⑪ My hands are numb.

⑫ My ankle still hurts me slightly.

⑬ My periods are somewhat irregular.

Right/Left/Both Body part + Do/Be 동사 + "Symptoms"

① Left side of my vision gets blurry.

② I have a pain on the right side of my head.

③ I have developed cataracts in both my eyes.

④ I started having chest pains on the left side of my chest.

⑤ My right arm is so sore.

⑥ My right ear has always hurt.

Words

bad cough: 심한 감기

a bad cut: 깊게 베인

indigestion: 소화불량

coughing up blood/bringing up blood: 객혈을 하다(피를 토하다)

can't catch my breath: 숨쉬기가 곤란하다

clogged up: 막히다(~가 막혀서/먹먹해서)

cataract(s): 백내장

period: 생리

periods: 생리주기

TIP

Irregular periods: 생리불순

(=) irregular cycles

(=) irregular menstrual cycle

Missed period: 생리를 건너뛴

Late period: 예정일 보다 늦은 생리

I initially had my period every fortnight about 3-4 times and then I did not have one for almost 60-70 days. : 나는 처음에 2주마다 생리를 3-4번 정도 하고 그 후로 거의 60-70일 동안 생리가 없었습니다.

Drill: 아래의 질문을 영작하세요

정답은 전 페이지의 Key Expressions을 참고하세요.

I have + "Symptoms."

Q1. 독감에 걸렸습니다.

____

Q2. 감기에 걸렸습니다.

____

Q3. 콧물이 흘러요.

____

Q4. 오한이 있어요.

____

Q5. 기침이 심해요.

____

Q6. 발진이 생겼어요.

____

Q7. 깊게 (칼에) 베었어요.

____

Q8. 속이 쓰려요.

____

Q9. 입안이 마릅니다.

____

Q10. 소화불량이에요.

____

Q11. 지난 2~3일 동안 설사를 해요.

____

Q12. 아침에 자주 코피가 나요.

____

Q13. 근육에 경련이 생겼어요.

____

Q14. 하루 종일 객혈을 해요.

____

Q15. 숨쉬기가 곤란해요.

____

I Do/Be 동사 + "Symptoms."

Q1. 온몸이 아파요.

____

Q2. 재채기를 심하게 해요.

____

Q3. 오심이 있어요.

____

Q4. 식욕이 전혀 없어요.

____

Q5. 숨쉬기가 곤란해요.

____

Q6. 하루 종일 어지러워요.

____

Q7. 최근에 걸린 감기 때문에 목이 쉬었어요.

____

Q8. 항상 피곤해요.

____

My ~ Do/Be 동사 + "Symptoms"

Q1. 눈이 가려워요.

____

Q2. 눈물이 많이 나와요.

____

Q3. 눈이 빛에 민감해요.

____

Q4. 뿌옇게(흐릿하게) 보여요.

____

Q5. 피부가 가려워요.

____

Q6. 입술이 텄어요.

____

Q7. 목이 따끔거리고 아파요.

____

Q8. 위가 아파요.

____

Q9. 귀가 먹먹해서 잘 안들려요.

____

Q10. 입이 마르고 까끌까끌 해요.

____

Q11. 손에 감각이 무뎌져요.

____

Q12. 발목이 여전히 아파요.

____

Q13. 생리주기가 다소 불규칙해요.

____

Right/Left/Both body part Do/Be 동사 + "Symptoms"

Q1. 왼쪽 눈이 흐릿하게 보여요.

____

Q2. 머리 오른쪽 부위가 아파요.

____

Q3. 양쪽 눈에 백내장이 생겼어요.

____

Q4. 왼쪽 흉부 부위에서 흉통을 느끼기 시작했어요.

____

Q5. 오른쪽 팔이 심하게 쑤셔요.

____

Q6. 오른쪽 귀가 항상 아파요.

____

Key Expressions: "~가 아프셔서 오셨나요?"

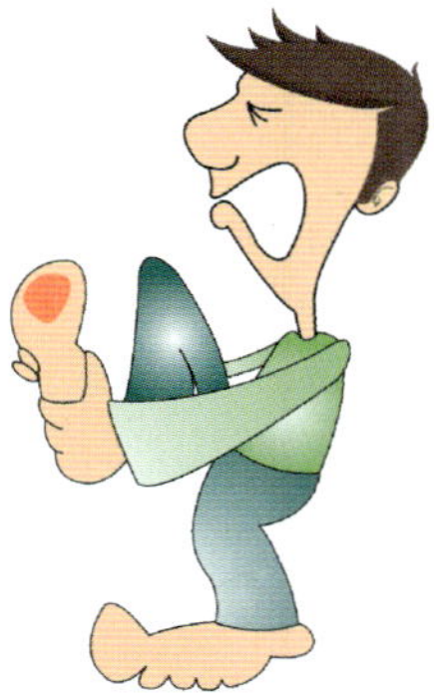

What~으로 시작하는 "~가 아프셔서 오셨나요?"

Q1. What brings you to my office today?

A1. I have terrible constipation.

Q2. What can I do for you today?

A2. I have swollen ankles.

Q3. What seems to be the problem?

A3. My cluster headaches are acting up again.

Q4. What's brought you along today?

A4. I think I've got the Flu.

Key Expressions: "~가 아프셔서 오셨나요?"

Q5. What's the nature of your visit?

A5. I feel much better after my treatment, but I still experience shortness of breath.

Q6. What seems to be the trouble with you, sir?

A6. I have been throwing up all day.

Q7. What made you come in today?

A7. I've got blotches all over my face.

How~로 시작하는 "~가 아프셔서 오셨나요?"

Q8. How can I help you?

A8. I have bloody diarrhea.

Q9. How have you been doing?

A9. I hear ringing in my ears.

Key Expressions: "~부위가 아프세요?"

Where/Which~로 시작하는 "~부위가 아프세요?"

Q10. Where does it hurt?

A10. I pulled my back.

Q11. Please show me where you feel the pain.

A11. It's right here under the rib cage.

Q12. Could you point out exactly where with your finger?

A12. Right here. (Point out your affected area with your finger.)

Q13. Where is the pain located?

A13. The pain is on the left side of my head.

Q14. Which part of your arm is sore?

A14. Sometimes my forearm is sore.

Words

acting up again: 재발하다, 악화되다

throw up: 토해요

blotch: 붉은 반점

pulled my back: 허리를 삐끗하다

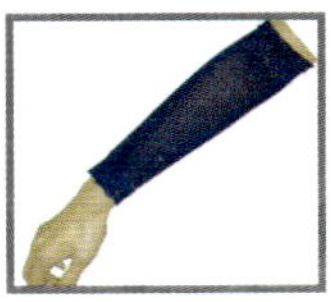

vs

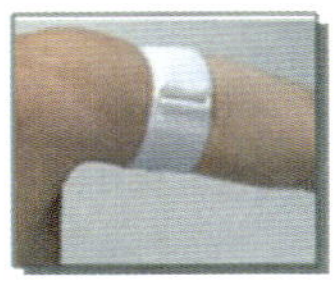

Forearm: 전완 Upper arm: 상완(팔뚝)

affected/affected area: 아픈 부위의

rib cage: 갈비뼈

sore: 쑤시다

Bed sore: 욕창

Canker sore: 구내염

Cold sore (=fever blisters): 입술포진

Drill: Q1-Q14 어디가 아프셔서 오셨습니까?의 표현을 영작하세요. Q15-Q28은 Fill in the blanks 문제입니다. 알맞은 구문을 넣어 완성하세요. 정답은 전 페이지의 Key Expressions를 참고하세요.

What~으로 시작하는 "~아프세요?"

Q1. 어디가 아프셔서 오셨습니까?

____

Q2. 어디가 아프세요?

____

Q3. 어디가 아프신가요?

____

Q4. 어디가 아프셔서 오셨습니까?

____

Q5. 어디가 아프셔서 오셨습니까?

____

Q6. 선생님, 어디가 아프세요?

____

Q7. 어디가 아프셔서 오셨나요?

____

How~로 시작하는 "~아프세요?"

Q 8. 어디가 아프세요?

____

Q9. 어디가 아프세요?

____

Where/Which~로 시작하는 "~아프세요?"

Q10. 어디가 아프세요?

____

Q11. 어디가 아픈지 보여주세요.

____

Q12. 정확하게 어디인지 손가락으로 가리켜 주시겠어요.

____

Q13. 어느 부위가 아픈가요?

____

Q14. 팔의 어느 부위가 아픈가요?

____.

Fill in the blanks

Q15. I have ______________________________.
나는 심한 변비가 있습니다.

Q16. I have______________________________.
발목이 부었습니다.

Q17. My____________________ are acting up again.
군집성 두통이 재발했어요.

Q18. I feel much better after my treatment, but I still experience______________________________.
치료받은 후 차도가 있긴 한데, 아직도 숨이 가쁩니다.

Q19. I think I've got______________________________.
독감에 걸린 것 같습니다.

Q20. Right here. (Point out your ____________with your finger.)
바로 여기요. (아픈 부위를 손가락으로 가리킨다.)

Q21. I have ______________________________.
피가 섞인 설사를 해요.

Q22. I have been ____________________ all day.
하루 종일 토해요.

Q23. I ____in my ears.

귀에서 소리가 들려요.

Q24. I've got ____________________________all over my face.

얼굴에 온통 붉은 반점이 생겼어요.

Q25. I ____my back.

허리를 삐끗했어요.

Q26. It's right here____________________________________.

갈비뼈 바로 아래쪽이요.

Q27. Sometimes my____________________________________.

때때로 나의 팔꿈치 아래가(전완) 아파요.

Q28. The pain is____.

머리 왼쪽 부위가 아파요.

3. Story of My Symptoms
나의 증상 이야기

- **Cold Sweat, 식은땀**

  - Words, 어휘

Story of My Symptoms

Cold Sweat

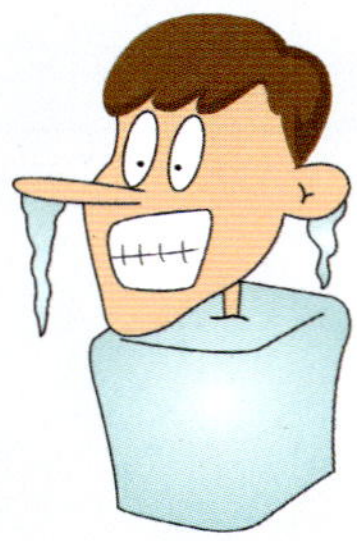

Question:

I keep waking up in a cold sweat.

I have been consistently waking up at night in a cold sweat for about six months. My health seems to be normal though, and this has never happened before, any ideas?

Answer:

The most common cause for the symptoms that you describe is stress. You do not mention whether this could indeed be a factor in your symptoms, but it would be worth looking at your lifestyle to see if there has been a recent build up of work or worry. Sometimes, there is no apparent cause for the symptoms that you describe and they are then described as 'idiopathic' and will often settle of their own accord over a period of time, but it is best to be certain so go and have a chat with your GP.

Yours sincerely,

The Medical Team

Words

keep waking: 계속해서 (잠에서) 깨다

consistently: 지속적으로

cold sweat: 식은땀

though: ~일지라도

common: 흔한

describe: 묘사하다, 설명하다

indeed: 정말로

be worth looking: ~할 가치가 있다

build up: 누적된, 과중 된

idiopathic: It means that the cause is unknown.
특발성 (질환)의: 원인을 알 수 없다는 의미이다.

settle of: 해결되다

their own accord: 그들 스스로

over a period of time: 시간이 지남에 따라

certain: 확실한

GP (General Practitioner): 일반의(사)

go and have a chat with your GP:
가서 당신의 일반의(사)와 상담을 하세요

Yours sincerely: 편지 글의 마지막 부분에 격식을 차려, ~ 올림

4. Frequently Asked Questions for My Symptoms 증상에 관해 자주하는 질문

A. FAQ for Constipation, 변비에 관해 자주하는 질문

- Words, 어휘
- Drill, 연습문제

B. FAQ for Appetite & Weight Changes, 식욕과 체중변화에 관해 자주하는 질문

- Words, 어휘
- Drill, 연습문제

C. FAQ for Temperature & Sweats, 발열과 발한에 관해 자주하는 질문

- Words, 어휘
- Drill, 연습문제

A. FAQ for Constipation

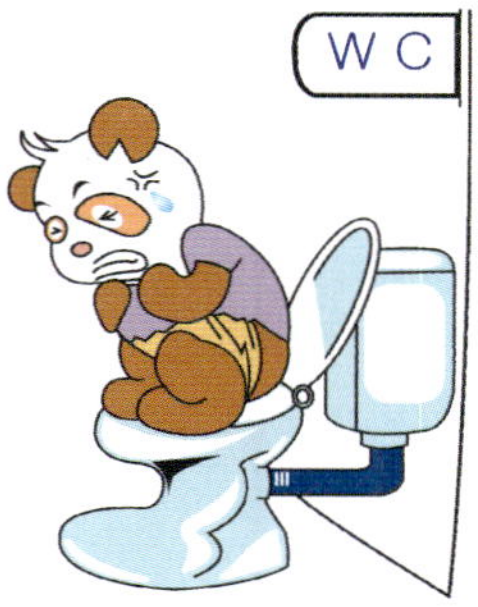

Q1. Are you suffering from chronic constipation?

A1. Yes. I have struggled with constipation all my life.

Q2. Are you currently taking any laxatives?

A2. Yes. I am taking Dulcolax to relieve my irregularity.

Q3. How many bowel movements do you have each day?

A3. I get bowel movements 3-4 times a day.

Q4. I feel terribly bloated. How can I relieve my constipation?

A4. I will prescribe something to relieve your constipation.

Q5. Do you suffer from irregularity?

A5. Yes. I suffer from irregularity. My tummy is distended and aching badly.

Words

irregularity (=constipation): 변비

laxative: 변비약

I feel terribly bloated.: 배가 너무 더부룩해요.

distended: 복부가 팽만한

badly: 심하게

Types of Laxatives: 변비약 종류

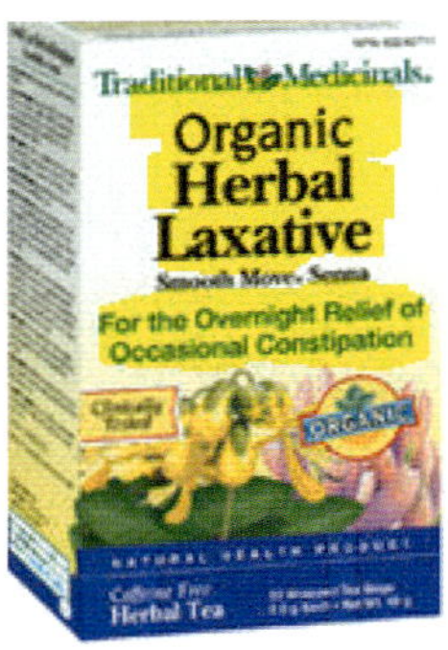

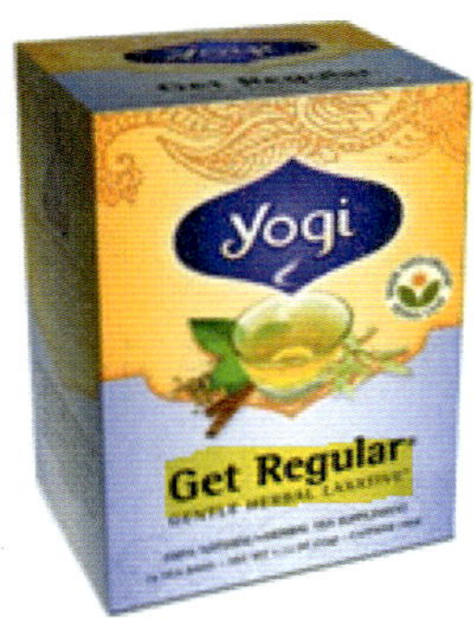

TIP

Get Regular: 규칙적으로 변을 보다.

Organic Herbal Laxative Tea: 변비를 완화시키는 유기농 차

Occasional Constipation: 일시적인 변비

Overnight Relief: 효과가 빠른

Drill: Q1-Q5는 Fill in the blanks 문제입니다. 알맞은 구문을 넣어 완성하세요. Q6-Q10의 FAQ를 영작하세요.

정답은 전 페이지의 FAQ를 참고하세요.

Fill in the blanks

Q1. I ______________________________all my life.

저는 평생 변비로 고생했습니다.

Q2. I am ________Dulcolax ______________________________.

변비를 완화시키기 위해 둘코락스를 복용하고 있습니다.

Q3. I get______________________________ 3-4 times a day.

하루에 서너 번 대변을 보기 위해 화장실에 갑니다.

Q4. I will prescribe something______________________________.

변비를 완화시킬 약을 처방해 드리겠습니다.

Q5. I ______________________________.

변비로 고생합니다.

My tummy is ____________ and ___________badly.

배가 더부룩하고 심하게 아파요.

FAQ

Q6. 만성변비로 고생하십니까?

Q7. 현재 변비약을 복용 중이신가요?

Q8. 하루에 화장실에 몇 번 가시나요?

Q9. 배가 너무 더부룩해요. 변비를 어떻게 완화시킬 수 있나요?

Q10. 변비로 고생하십니까?

B. FAQ for Appetite & Weight Changes

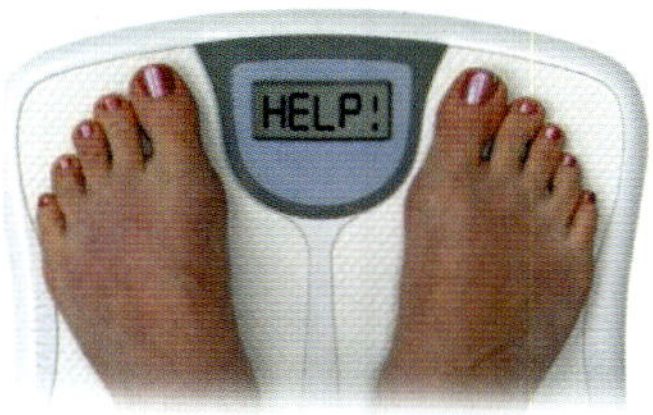

Q1. Have you noticed any weight changes lately?

A1. Yes. I have lost more than 6 kilograms over the past two months.

Q2. Have you gained or lost weight?

A2. Yes. Recently, I have been gaining weight really fast.

Q3. How is your appetite?

A3. Well, I used to have a great appetite, but I don't have much of an appetite nowadays.

Q4. Are you on a diet?

A4. Yes. I am always on a diet to lose weight.

Q5. Have you ever had episodes of eating a large amount of food in a very short time?

A5. Yes. I have gone on binges where I felt I could not stop eating.

Words

diet pill: 살 빼는 약

great appetite: 식욕이 왕성한

on a diet: 다이어트 중

episodes of: 발병했던 적

binge: 폭식(섭식장애의 일종)

TIP

Eating disorder: 섭식장애

Anorexia Nervosa: 거식증

Bulimia Nervosa: 폭식증(식욕이상 항진증: 음식을 폭식하고 토해내기를 반복하는 증세)

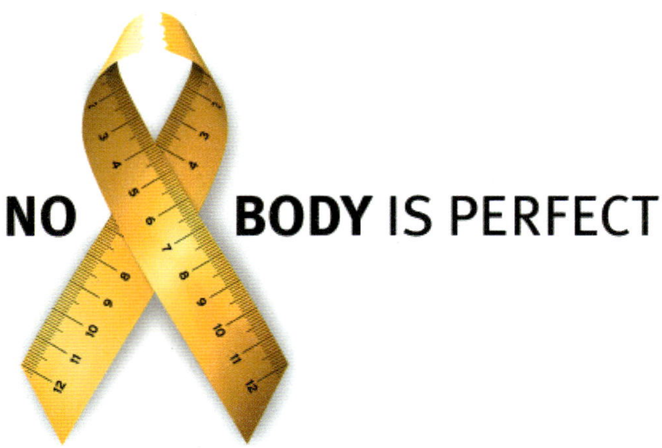

bingeeatingdisorder-help.com

Drill: Q1-Q5는 Fill in the blanks 문제입니다. 알맞은 구문을 넣어 완성하세요. Q6-Q10의 FAQ를 영작하세요.
정답은 전 페이지의 FAQ를 참고하세요.

Fill in the blanks

Q1. I ________________________over the past two months.
지난 2개월 동안 6 킬로그램 이상이 빠졌습니다.

Q2. Recently, I have been_____________________________.
최근에 갑작스럽게 체중이 늘었습니다.

Q3. I used to have____________________, but I don't have _____________nowadays.
예전에는 식욕이 왕성했으나 요즘은 식욕이 없습니다.

Q4. I am always_____________________________________.
저는 살을 빼기 위해 항상 다이어트 중입니다.

Q5. I have gone _____________where I felt I could not stop eating.
음식을 멈출 수 없을 정도로 폭식을 한 적이 있습니다.

FAQ

Q6. 최근에 체중의 변화가 있습니까?

____

Q7. 체중이 늘거나 또는 줄었나요?

____

Q8. 식욕은 어떤가요?

____

Q9. 다이어트 중인가요?

____

Q10. 아주 짧은 시간에 많은 양의 음식을 섭취한 적이 있습니까?

____

C. FAQ for Temperature & Sweats

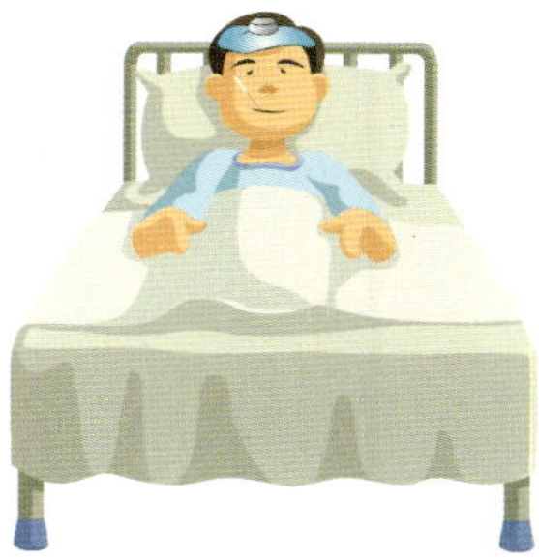

Q1. Do you feel feverish?/Do you have a fever?

A1. Yes. I am running a high fever.

Q2. Do you wake up in a cold sweat at night?

A2. Yes. I wake up in a cold sweat at least three times a week.

Q3. Do you sweat a lot?

A3. Yes. I am always soaked in sweat.

Q4. Are you having chills?

A4. Yes. I get the chills.

Q5. Are you suffering from night sweats?

A5. Yes. I literally drench my bed with sweat at night.

Words

feverish: 열이 나는

cold sweat: 식은땀

soaked in sweat: 땀에 흠뻑 젖은

chills: 오한

drench: ~ 흠뻑 젖은

night sweats: 밤에 땀을 많이 흘리는 증상

TIP

Symptoms of Menopause: 폐경기증상

Night sweats: 밤에 땀을 많이 흘림

Hot flashes: 안면 홍조

The first symptoms of menopause are night sweats and hot flashes. : 폐경기에 우선적으로 나타나는 증상은 밤에 땀을 많이 흘리는 증상과 안면 홍조이다.

Drill: Q1-Q5는 Fill in the blanks 문제입니다. 알맞은 구문을 넣어 완성하세요. Q6-Q10의 FAQ를 영작하세요.
정답은 전 페이지의 FAQ를 참고하세요.

Fill in the blanks

Q1. I am ______________________________.
고열이 납니다.

Q2. I wake up ____________at least three times a week.
일주일에 적어도 3번은 식은땀을 흘리며 깹니다.

Q3. I am always______________________________.
항상 땀을 아주 많이 흘립니다.

Q4. I get______________________________.
오한이 납니다.

Q5. I literally ______________________at night.
말 그대로 밤에 잘 때 침대가 땀에 흠뻑 젖어요.

FAQ

Q6. 열이 있나요?

Q7. 한밤중에 식은땀을 흘리며 잠에서 깨나요?

Q8. 땀을 많이 흘리나요?

Q9. 오한이 나요?

Q10. 밤에 땀을 많이 흘리나요?

5. Describing My Symptoms
나의 증상 설명하기

A. Constipation, 변비

- Dialogue, 대화
- Words, 어휘
- Anatomy: GI Tract, 인체이야기: 위장관
- Review, 복습
- Pop Quiz, 퀴즈

B. Chest Pain & Dizzy Spells, 흉통과 어지러움

- Dialogue, 대화
- Words, 어휘
- Anatomy: The Structure of the Heart, 인체이야기: 심장 구조
- Review, 복습
- Pop Quiz, 퀴즈

C. Stiff and Aching Knee Joints, 뻣뻣하고 아픈 무릎관절

- Dialogue, 대화
- Words, 어휘
- Anatomy: Structure of the Knee, 인체이야기: 무릎 구조
- Review, 복습
- Pop Quiz, 퀴즈

D. Concerns about My Eyes, 아픈 눈

- Dialogue, 대화
- Words, 어휘
- Anatomy: The Structure of the Eye, 인체이야기: 눈 구조
- Review, 복습
- Pop Quiz, 퀴즈

Describing My Symptoms

A. Constipation

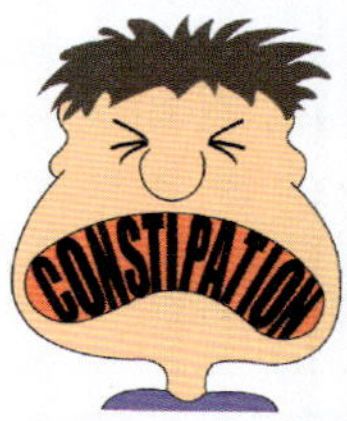

Doctor: Have you noticed any appetite changes recently?

Patient: Yes. I have lost my appetite.

Doctor: I see. Is your bowel movement regular?

Patient: It was, but not anymore.

Doctor: When was your last bowel movement?

Patient: About 4 days ago.

Doctor: Do you have any other symptoms that occur with constipation?

Patient: Um. I suffer from gas, so I feel so bloated. On top of that, I feel nauseous, too.

Doctor: I see. Are you currently taking any medications to relieve your discomforts?

Patient: Yes. But it won't work for me.

Doctor: I am going to examine your belly. Please get on the examination table.

Words

lose my appetite: 식욕을 잃다

gas: 가스가 차다

bloated: 복부가 팽만한

feel nauseous: 메스껍습니다

bowel movement(s): 배변(배변을 보는 것)

examination table: 검사대

TIP

Belly, Tummy, Abdomen: 복부

Belly button, Navel: 배꼽

Anatomy: GI Tract

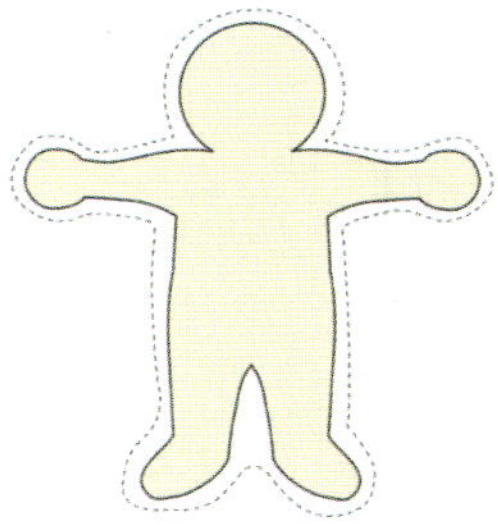

Esophagus: 식도

Stomach: 위

Liver: 간

Gall Bladder: 쓸개

Pancreas: 췌장

Large Intestine: 대장

Small Intestine: 소장

Appendix: 충수

Rectum: 직장

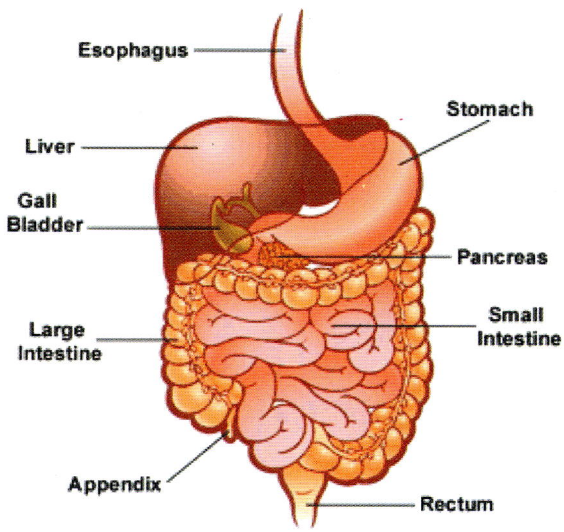

Review: 각각의 구문을 영작하세요.

정답은 전 페이지의 Dialogue를 참고하세요.

Doctor: 요즘 식욕에 변화가 있으신가요?

____

Patient: 예. 식욕이 없습니다.

____

Doctor: 알겠습니다. 변이 규칙적인가요?

____

Patient: It was, but not anymore.

Doctor: 언제 마지막으로 화장실에 가셨습니까?

____

Patient: About 4 days ago.

Doctor: 변비에 따른 다른 증상도 있습니까?

____

Patient: 음. 가스가 차서 고생해요. 가스가 상당히 많이 차요.

____

게다가, 속도 메스껍습니다.

____

Doctor: 알겠습니다. 현재 지금 증세를 완화시키는 약을 복용 중입니까?

Patient: Yes. But it won't work for me.

Doctor: I am going to examine your belly. Please get on the examination table.

Pop Quiz: Identify the part of the GI Tract indicated by an arrow. There are 9 questions in total.

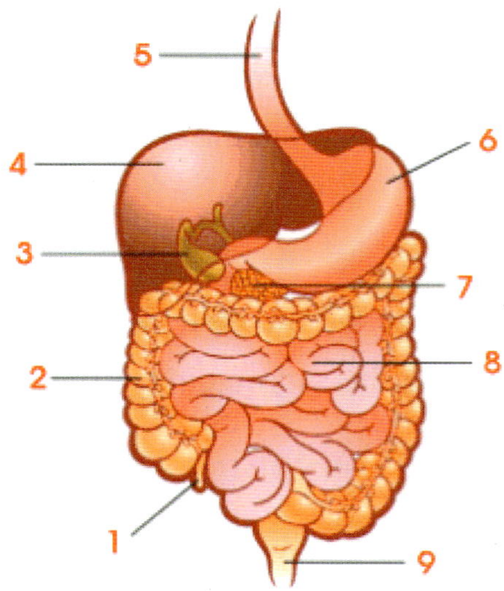

Describing My Symptoms

B. Chest Pain & Dizzy Spells

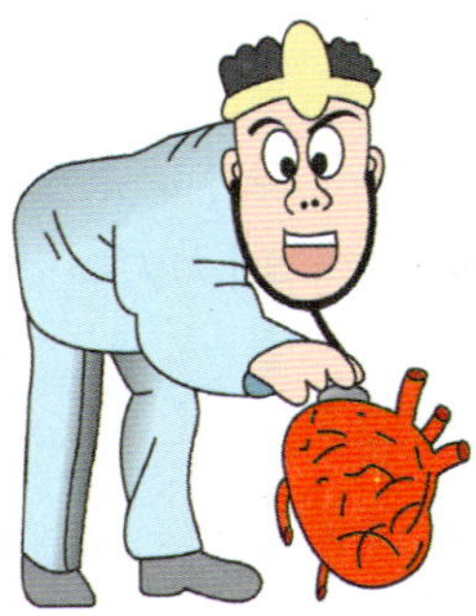

Doctor: Could you tell me what you are mostly concerned about?
Patient: Yes. My heart is pounding badly.

Doctor: I see. When did it first start?
Patient: I think it started last Tuesday.

Doctor: Do you feel the pain on the left side of your neck, shoulder, arm, or in your chest when you work out?
Patient: I think sometimes I feel the pain in my chest after exercise.

Doctor: Could you describe the pain, please?
Patient: Sure. It feels like something is squeezing me around my chest area.

Doctor: Have you had a similar episode in the past?
Patient: Yes. I had this around a month ago.

Doctor: Do you have any other symptoms that occur with it?
Patient: I think I have dizzy spells as well.

Doctor: Has anyone in your family suffered from similar conditions?
Patient: Not that I know of. Do you have any idea what's going on with me?

Doctor: I have some thoughts, but first we need to run some tests.
Patient: I hope it won't be serious.

Words

badly: 매우, 심하게

work out: 운동하다

squeezing: 꽉 조이는 듯한

episode: 질병의 발생

have dizzy spells: 어지럼증을 느껴요

run some tests: 몇 가지 검사를 하다

Anatomy: The Structure of the Heart

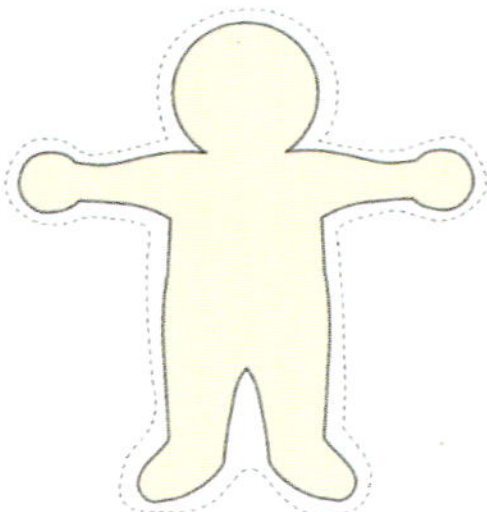

Superior Vena Cava: 상대정맥

Inferior Vena Cava: 하대정맥

Right Atrium: 우심방

Right Ventricle: 우심실

Pulmonary Artery: 폐동맥

Pulmonary Vein: 폐정맥

Left Atrium: 좌심방

Left Ventricle: 좌심실

Aortic Valve: 대동맥판

Aorta: 대동맥

Pulmonary Valve: 폐동맥판

Mitral Valve:

이첨판, 승모판

Tricuspid Valve:

삼첨판

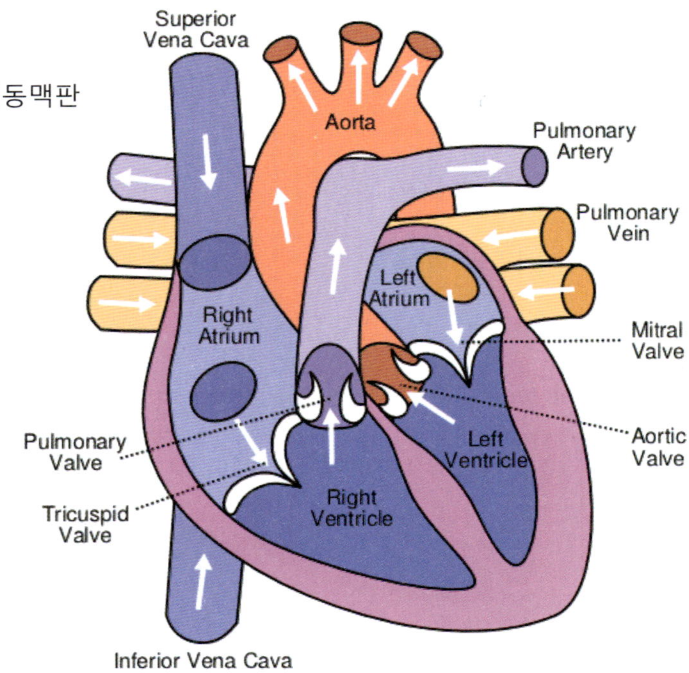

Review: 각각의 구문을 영작하세요.
정답은 전 페이지의 Dialogue를 참고하세요.

Doctor: 가장 염려되시는 것이 무엇인지 말씀해 주시겠습니까?

____

Patient: Yes. My heart is pounding badly.

Doctor: 알겠습니다. 처음 시작된 때가 언제인가요?

____

Patient: I think it started last Tuesday.

Doctor: 운동을 할 때 왼쪽 목, 어깨, 팔 또는 가슴에 통증을 느끼나요?

____

Patient: I think sometimes I feel the pain in my chest after exercise.

Doctor: 통증을 설명해 주시겠습니까?

____

Patient: Sure. It feels like something is squeezing me around my chest area.

Doctor: 전에도 이런 적이 있었습니까?

____

Patient: Yes. I had this around a month ago.

Doctor: 다른 증상도 있나요?

____

Patient: I think, I have dizzy spells as well.

Doctor: 가족 중에 비슷한 증상으로 아픈 사람이 있나요?

____

Patient: Not that I know of. Do you have any idea what's going on with me?

Doctor: 내 소견에 앞서 먼저 몇 가지 검사를 하겠습니다.

____

Patient: I hope it won't be serious.

Pop Quiz: Identify the part of the heart indicated by an arrow. There are 9 questions in total.

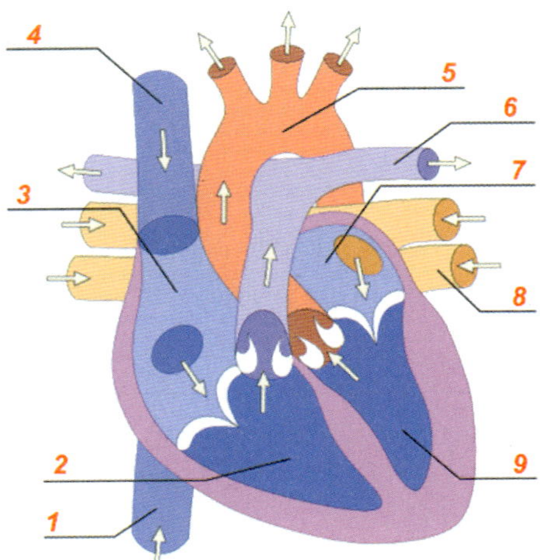

Describing My Symptoms

C. Stiff and Aching Knee Joints

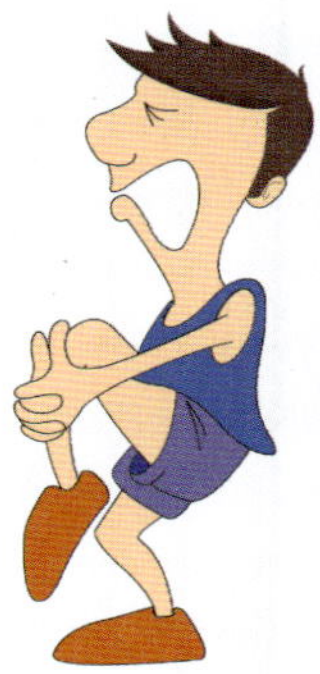

Doctor: So, we have several things going on here. Let's talk about your knee first. Can you describe your pain please?

Patient: Well, my knee joints are very stiff and aching.

Doctor: When did you first notice the pain?

Patient: Well, it started two weeks ago.

Doctor: How bad is your pain?

Patient: It is severely painful.

Doctor: Is it worse at a certain time of the day?

Patient: Yes. It gets worse at night, and it's so unbearable.

Doctor: Is there anything that makes you feel better when you are in pain?

Patient: I haven't found any cures yet. Even the pain medications won't work.

Doctor: Well, I'd like to run some tests including blood work. Also, I need to take X-rays of your knees.

Patient: I see.

Words

knee joints: 무릎관절

stiff: 뻣뻣한

severely: 심하게

get worse: 더 악화되다

blood work: 혈액검사

take X-rays of ~: ~ 엑스레이를 찍다

Anatomy: The Structure of the Knee

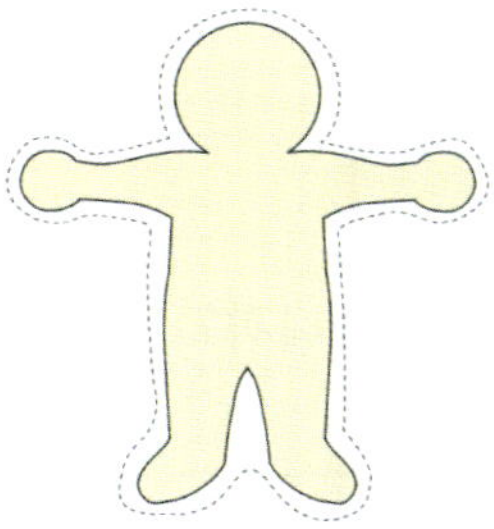

Femur: 대퇴골

Patella: 슬개골

Tibia: 경골

Anterior Cruciate Ligament (ACL): 전방십자인대

Posterior Cruciate Ligament: 후방십자인대

Medial ligament: 내측인대

Lateral ligament: 외측인대

Meniscus: 반월상 연골

Lateral meniscus: 외측 반월상 연골

Medial meniscus: 내측 반월상 연골

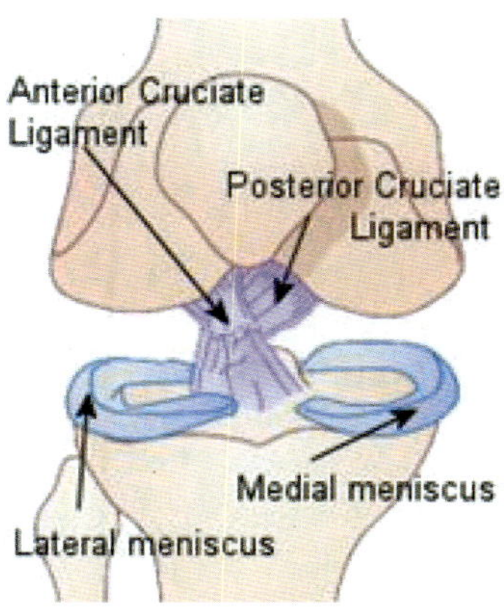

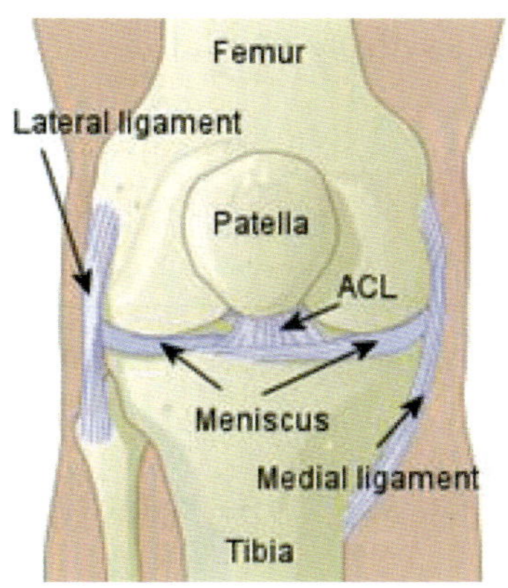

Review: 각각의 구문을 영작하세요.

정답은 전 페이지의 Dialogue를 참고하세요.

Doctor: So, we have several things going on here.

무릎부터 먼저 시작하겠습니다. 통증에 대해 설명해 주시겠습니까?

Patient: 무릎관절이 뻣뻣하고 아파요.

Doctor: 처음 통증을 느낀 시기가 언제 인가요?

Patient: Well, it started two weeks ago.

Doctor: 통증이 얼마나 심한가요?

Patient: It is severely painful.

Doctor: 하루 중 어느 특정한 때에 통증이 더 악화되나요?

Patient: Yes. It gets worse at night, and it's so unbearable.

Doctor: 통증을 완화시키는 것이 있습니까?

Patient: I haven't found any cures yet. Even the pain medications won't work.

Doctor: 음. 혈액검사를 포함한 몇 가지 검사를 하겠습니다.

또한, 무릎 엑스레이도 찍겠습니다.

Patient: I see.

Pop Quiz: Identify the part of the knee indicated by an arrow. There are 8 questions in total.

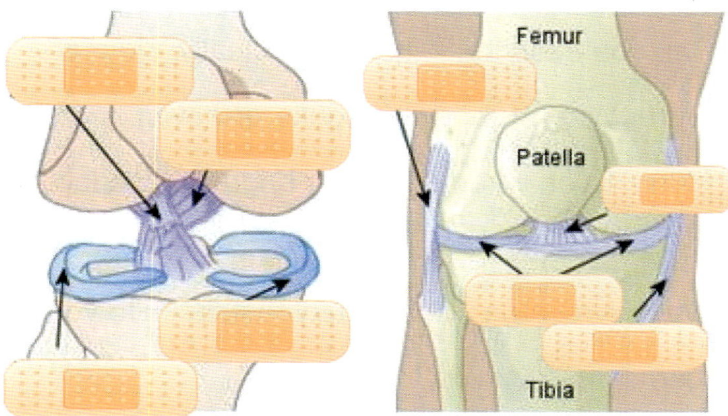

Describing My Symptoms

D. Concerns about My Eyes

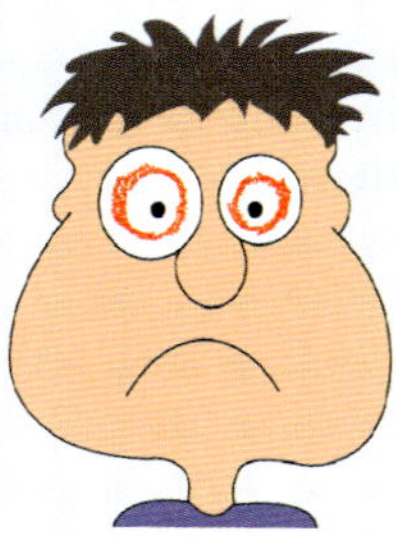

Doctor: What seems to be the trouble with you, ma'am?

Patient: Um. I think my vision has decreased. Sometimes, I'm not able to see clearly what is in front of me.

Doctor: Can you describe it more specifically, please?

Patient: Sure. When I read the books or newspaper, the letters are very blurry. Even when there is a bright light, it looks dim.

Doctor: We'll give you a visual acuity test first. Do you have any other concerns in your mind?

Patient: Yes. I noticed a sudden increase in the number of floaters in my right eye. Also, my eyes also seem to be more light sensitive lately.

Doctor: I see. I need to check your eye pressure and do several other eye exams to determine the cause of these conditions.

Patient: Is it serious?

Doctor: We'll talk about it after the tests.

Words

vision: 시력

dim: 희미하게 보임

visual acuity test: 시력 검사

floaters: 날파리증/비문증(눈앞에 먼지나 벌레 같은 것이 떠다니는 느낌)

light sensitive: 빛에 민감한

eye pressure: 안압

Chapter 4

Anatomy: The Structure of the Eye

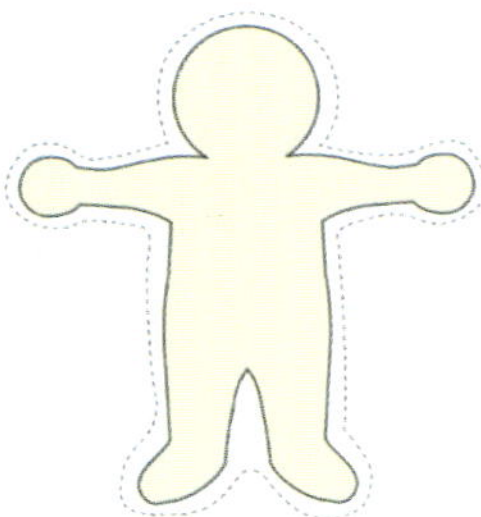

Sclera: 공막(흰자위)

Iris: 홍채

Pupil: 동공

Cornea: 각막

Lens: 수정체

Posterior Capsule: 수정체낭 후막

Retina: 망막

Macula: 황반

Optic Nerve: 시신경

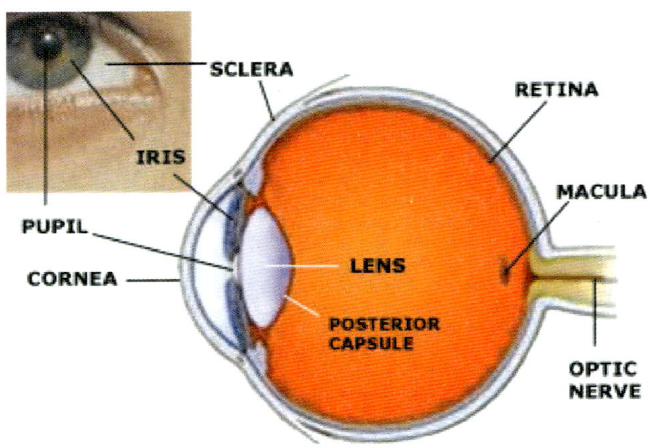

Review: 각각의 구문을 영작하세요.

정답은 전 페이지의 Dialogue를 참고하세요.

Doctor: What seems to be the trouble with you, ma'am?

Patient: 음. 내 생각에 시력이 나빠진 것 같아요.

때때로 내 앞에 있는 것도 잘 안보입니다.

Doctor: Can you describe it more specifically, please?

Patient: 예. 내가 책이나 신문을 읽을 때, 글자가 또렷해 보이지 않아요.

Even when there is a bright light, it looks dim.

Doctor: We'll give you a visual acuity test first.

다른 염려 사항이 있습니까?

Patient: 예. 오른쪽 눈에 먼지 같고 작은 벌레 같은 것들이 떠다니는 것 같은 부유물들이 갑자기 더 많아 졌어요.

또한 최근에 제 눈이 빛에 더 민감해진 것 같습니다.

Doctor: 알겠습니다. 이러한 증상들의 원인을 알기 위해 안압 검사와 몇 가지 눈검사가 필요합니다.

Patient: Is it serious?

Doctor: We'll talk about it after the tests.

Pop Quiz: Identify the part of the Eye indicated by an arrow. There are 7 questions in total.

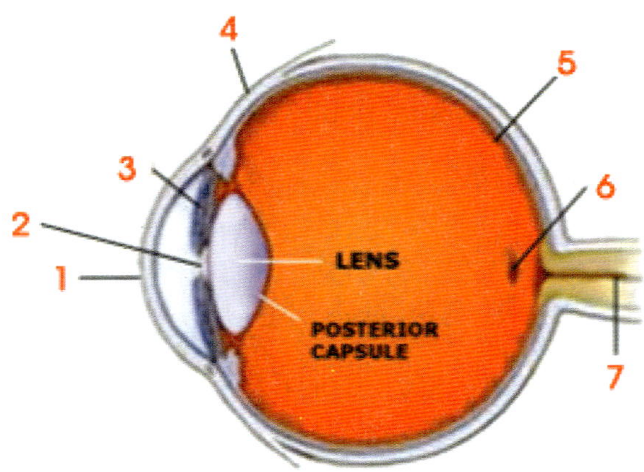

6. Reading Material
독해구문

· **Springtime Allergy, 계절성 앨러지**

- Words, 어휘

Reading Material

Springtime Allergy

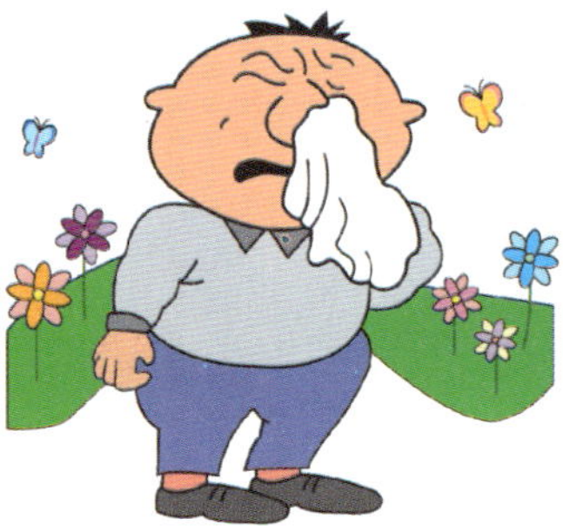

Spring means flower buds and blooming trees — and if you're one of the millions of people who have springtime allergies, it also means sneezing, congestion, runny nose and other bothersome symptoms.

Springtime allergies — also called hay fever and allergic rhinitis — can make you miserable. But before you settle for plastic flowers and artificial turf, try these simple strategies to keep springtime allergies under control.

Reduce your exposure to allergy triggers

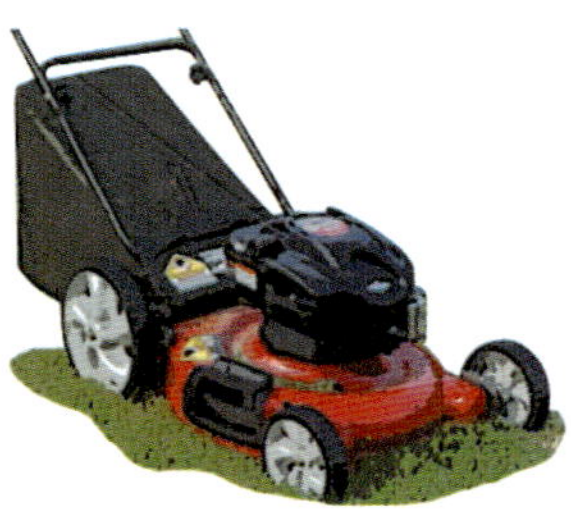

There are a number of things that you can do to reduce your exposure to the things that trigger your allergy signs and symptoms (allergens):

- Stay indoors on dry, windy days — the best time to go outside is after a good rain, which helps clear pollen from the air.
- Delegate lawn mowing, weed pulling and other gardening chores that stir up allergens.
- Remove clothes you've worn outside; you may also want to shower to rinse pollen from your skin and hair.
- Don't hang laundry outside — pollen can stick to sheets and towels.
- Wear a dust mask if you do outside chores.

Take extra steps when pollen counts are high

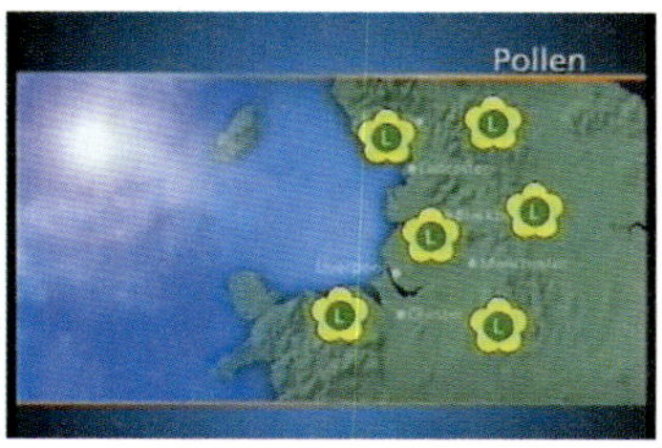

Seasonal allergy signs and symptoms can flare up when there's a lot of pollen in the air. These steps can help you reduce your exposure:

- Check your local TV or radio station, your local newspaper, or the Internet for pollen forecasts and current pollen levels.
- If high pollen counts are forecasted, start taking allergy medications before your symptoms start.
- Close doors and windows at night or any other time when pollen counts are high.
- Avoid outdoor activity in the early morning when pollen counts are the highest.

Source: Mayoclinic staff

Words

sneezing: 재채기

congestion: 코 막힘

runny nose: 콧물

bothersome: 고통스러운

hay fever: 꽃가루 앨러지

allergic rhinitis: 앨러지성 비염

artificial turf: 인공잔디

allergens: 앨러지 유발인자

a good rain: 비가 흠뻑 온

delegate: (다른 사람에게) ~을 위임하세요

lawn mowing: 잔디 깎는 일

weed pulling: 잡초(민들레) 뽑는 일, 미국에서는 민들레도 잡초의 일종

gardening chores: 정원 일

pollen counts: 꽃가루 수치

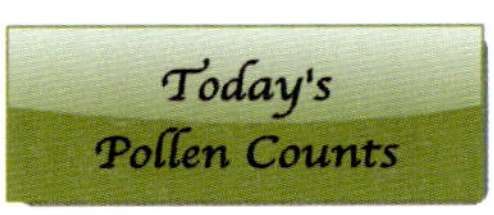

오늘의 꽃가루 수치

6. 해석 및 정답

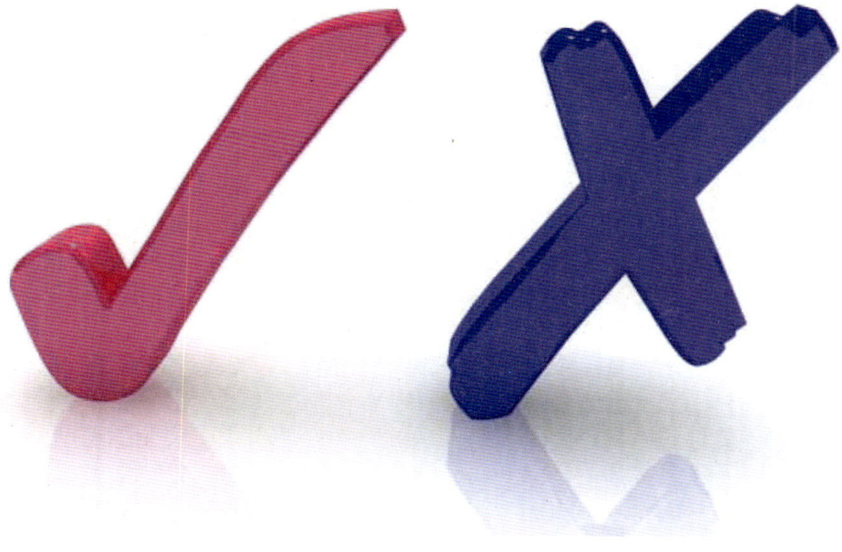

1. 증상의 종류

주요어휘: 주요어휘 연습문제

G. 빈혈

왼쪽은 빈혈환자의 창백한 손 오른쪽은 내과의사 선생님 손

C	Q	N	C	H	I	L	L	S	Q	N	M	L	U	Q	U	P
Y	O	Q	U	E	A	S	Y	S	R	R	O	E	S	X	F	I
A	G	L	B	A	D	F	M	H	E	A	R	T	B	U	R	N
N	Q	Q	D	T	E	I	R	Q	D	W	N	H	A	P	G	K
O	Y	N	P		R	O	Z	B	I	K	I	A	A	S	B	Y
S	B	C	I	R	S	I	W	Z	X	U	N	R	W	E	S	
I	M	B	I	A	S	W	H	N	Y	M	G	G	T	A	E	E
S	B	H	J	S	I	K	E	P	Y			Y	O	S	F	Y
B	Q	A	C	H	L	H	E	A	T		S	T	R	O	K	E
G	N	T	B	J	I	Q	Z	L	T	A	T	P	L	N	P	S
H	G	L	W	V	Y	P	E	L	L	J	I	F	E	A	Y	N
W	T	K	E	N	J	W	P	O	K	E	F	R	Q	L	N	L
D	A	S	X	I	J	X	V	R	K	A	F	W	I		L	A
N	W	S	T	S	Q	K	O	S	R	S	N	X	C	F	X	S
M	T	W	I	T	C	H	I	N	G		E	Y	E	L	I	D
K	N	C	Y	W	P	Q	E	O	F	O	S	J	G	U	S	B
X	O	J	X	Q	L	T	R	J	Q	K	S	Q	W	Y	H	J

Lethargy	Heartburn	Queasy
Wheeze	Cold sweat	Chills
Seasonal flu	Morning stiffness	Heat rash
		Hives
Pallor	Pinky eyes	Twitching eyelid
Dizzy spells	Heat stroke	Cyanosis

1. 증상의 종류

J. 유아질환 관련 증상: 주요어휘 연습문제

D	M	X	Y	L	F	J	N	K	B	U	M	R	P	H
Q	M	I	S	N	X	E	T	T	G	G	B	A	G	A
U	B	U	M	V	G	O	V	H	U	T	Q	P	C	Q
O	Q	L	V	A	T	X	I	E	N	R	Q	I	C	M
B	T	F	O	I	W	M	Y	F	R	M	E	D	J	E
G	R	U	N	T	I	N	G	A	E	L	X		G	D
P	U	W	P	M	C	G	S	Q	S	K	T	B	D	R
J	D	V	U	S	Q	H	P	R	P	A	G	R	U	I
P	B	Q	R	G	G	P	Y	N	O	M	O	E	R	S
Y	T	W	Q	Q	W	T	N		N	W	C	A	Q	N
E	D	L	I	S	T	L	E	S	S	P	O	T	S	G
E	C	G	R	F	A	R	S	Y	I	K	N	H	A	F
P	H	O	N	L	R	J	V	X	V	Q	I	I	Q	N
O	K	Q	S	H	V	P	J	S	E	W	B	N	C	A
N	J	C	G	E	V	O	M	I	T	I	N	G	T	N

Vomiting	Blotchy skin	Fever
Grunting	Spots	Rash
Listless	Unresponsive	Drowsy
Rapid breathing		

1. 증상의 종류
증상표현 주요구문 모음

I have "symptoms."

① 독감에 걸렸습니다.

② 감기에 걸렸습니다.

③ 콧물이 흘러요.

④ 오한이 있어요.

⑤ 기침이 심해요.

⑥ 발진이 생겼어요.

⑦ 깊게 (칼에) 베었어요.

⑧ 속이 쓰려요.

⑨ 입안이 마릅니다.

⑩ 소화불량이에요.

⑪ 지난 2~3일 동안 설사를 해요.

⑫ 아침에 자주 코피가 나요.

⑬ 근육에 경련이 생겼어요.

⑭ 하루 종일 객혈을 해요.

⑮ 숨쉬기가 곤란해요.

I Do/Be 동사 + "Symptoms."

① 온몸이 아파요.

② 재채기를 심하게 해요.

③ 오심이 있어요.

④ 식욕이 전혀 없어요.

⑤ 숨쉬기가 곤란해요.

⑥ 하루 종일 어지러워요.

⑦ 최근에 걸린 감기 때문에 목이 쉬었어요.

⑧ 항상 피곤해요.

My ~ Do/Be 동사 + "Symptoms"

① 눈이 가려워요.

② 눈물이 많이 나와요.

③ 눈이 빛에 민감해요.

④ 뿌옇게(흐릿하게) 보여요.

⑤ 피부가 가려워요.

⑥ 입술이 텄어요.

⑦ 목이 따끔거리고 아파요.

⑧ 위가 아파요.

⑨ 귀가 먹먹해서 잘 안 들려요.

⑩ 입이 마르고 까끌까끌 해요.

⑪ 손에 감각이 무뎌져요.

⑫ 발목이 여전히 아파요.

⑬ 생리주기가 다소 불규칙해요.

Right/Left/Both body part Do/Be 동사 + "Symptoms"

① 왼쪽 눈이 흐릿하게 보여요.

② 머리 오른쪽 부위가 아파요.

③ 양쪽 눈에 백내장이 생겼어요.

④ 왼쪽 흉부 부위에서 흉통을 느끼기 시작했어요.

⑤ 오른쪽 팔이 심하게 쑤셔요.

⑥ 오른쪽 귀가 항상 아파요.

2. 증상표현 주요구문 모음

주요구문

What~으로 시작하는 "~가 아프셔서 오셨나요?"

Q1. 어디가 아프셔서 오셨습니까?

A1. 나는 심한 변비가 있습니다.

Q2. 어디가 아프세요?

A2. 발목이 부었습니다.

Q3. 어디가 아프신가요?

A3. 군집성 두통이 재발했어요.

Q4. 어디가 아프셔서 오셨습니까?

A4. 독감에 걸린 것 같습니다.

Q5. 어디가 아프셔서 오셨습니까?

A5. 치료받은 후 차도가 있긴 한데, 아직도 숨이 가쁩니다.

Q6. 선생님, 어디가 아프세요?

A6. 하루 종일 토해요.

Q7. 어디가 아프셔서 오셨나요?

A7. 얼굴에 온통 붉은 반점이 생겼어요.

How~로 시작하는 "~가 아프셔서 오셨나요?"

Q8. 어디가 아프세요?

A8. 피가 섞인 설사를 해요.

Q9. 어디가 아프세요?

A9. 귀에서 소리가 들려요.

Where/Which~로 시작하는 "~부위가 아프세요?"

Q10. 어디가 아프세요?

A10. 허리를 삐끗했어요.

Q11. 어디가 아픈지 보여주세요.

A11. 갈비뼈 바로 아래쪽이요.

Q12. 정확하게 어디인지 손가락으로 가리켜 주시겠어요.

A12. 바로 여기요. (아픈 부위를 손가락으로 가리킨다.)

Q13. 어느 부위가 아픈가요?

A13. 머리 왼쪽 부위가 아파요.

Q14. 팔의 어느 부위가 아픈가요?

A14. 때때로 나의 팔꿈치 아래가(전완) 아파요.

3. 나의 증상 이야기
식은땀

질문: 저는 계속해서 식은 땀을 흘리며 깨어납니다.

나는 약 6개월 동안 지속적으로 밤 중에 식은 땀을 흘리며 깨어납니다. 그렇더라도 나의 건강은 정상인 듯 보이며, 전에는 이런 일이 일어난 적이 결코 없습니다.
좋은 고견이 있으십니까?

답변:

당신이 호소한 그 증상의 가장 흔한 원인은 스트레스입니다. 당신은 이것이(스트레스) 정말로 당신 증상의 원인인지 아닌지를 언급하지는 않았으나 최근에 가중된 업무 또는 걱정거리가 있는지의 여부를 알기 위해 당신의 삶을 살펴볼 필요가 있습니다. 때때로, 당신이 설명한 증상들에는 명백한 원인이 없고 '특발성'으로 설명되며 시간이 지남에 따라 저절로 해결됩니다. 하지만, 확실히 해두는 것이 최선이기에 당신의 의사선생님에게 가서 상의해 보세요.
의료팀 올림

4. 증상에 관해 자주하는 질문
변비에 관해 자주하는 질문

Q1. 만성변비로 고생하십니까?

A1. 예. 저는 평생 변비로 고생했습니다.

Q2. 현재 변비약을 복용 중이신가요?

A2. 예. 변비를 완화시키기 위해 둘코락스를 복용하고 있습니다.

Q3. 하루에 화장실에 몇 번 가시나요?

A3. 하루에 서너 번 대변을 보기 위해 화장실에 갑니다.

Q4. 배가 너무 더부룩해요. 변비를 어떻게 완화시킬 수 있나요?

A4. 변비를 완화시킬 약을 처방해 드리겠습니다.

Q5. 변비로 고생하십니까?

A5. 예. 변비로 고생합니다. 배가 더부룩하고 심하게 아파요.

4. 증상에 관해 자주하는 질문
식욕과 체중변화에 관해 자주하는 질문

Q1. 최근에 체중의 변화가 있습니까?

A1. 예, 지난 2개월 동안 6 킬로그램 이상이 빠졌습니다.

Q2. 체중이 늘거나 또는 줄었나요?

A2. 예, 최근에 갑작스럽게 체중이 늘었습니다.

Q3. 식욕은 어떤가요?

A3. 음, 예전에는 식욕이 왕성했으나 요즘은 식욕이 없습니다.

Q4. 다이어트 중인가요?

A4. 예, 저는 살을 빼기 위해 항상 다이어트 중입니다.

Q5. 아주 짧은 시간에 많은 양의 음식을 섭취한 적이 있습니까?

A5. 네. 음식을 멈출 수 없을 정도로 폭식을 한 적이 있습니다.

4. 증상에 관해 자주하는 질문
발열과 발한에 관해 자주하는 질문

Q1. 열이 있나요?

A1. 예. 고열이 납니다.

Q2. 한밤중에 식은땀을 흘리며 잠에서 깨나요?

A2. 예. 일주일에 적어도 3번은 식은땀을 흘리며 깹니다.

Q3. 땀을 많이 흘리나요?

A3. 예. 항상 땀을 아주 많이 흘립니다.

Q4. 오한이 나요?

A4. 예. 오한이 납니다.

Q5. 밤에 땀을 많이 흘리나요?

A5. 예. 말 그대로 밤에 잘 때 침대가 땀에 흠뻑 젖어요.

5. 나의 증상 설명하기

A. 변비

Doctor: 요즘 식욕에 변화가 있으신가요?

Patient: 예. 식욕이 없습니다.

Doctor: 알겠습니다. 변이 규칙적인가요?

Patient: 예전에는 규칙적이었으나 지금은 더 이상 아닙니다.

Doctor: 언제 마지막으로 화장실에 가셨습니까?

Patient: 약 4일전이요.

Doctor: 변비에 따른 다른 증상도 있습니까?

Patient: 음. 가스가 차서 고생해요. 가스가 상당히 많이 차요. 게다가, 속도 메스껍습니다.

Doctor: 알겠습니다. 현재 지금 증세를 완화시키는 약을 복용 중입니까?

Patient: 예. 하지만 약이 듣지 않습니다.

Doctor: 복부를 진찰하겠습니다. 검사 테이블에 올라와 주세요.

5. 나의 증상 설명하기

B. 흉통과 어지러움

Doctor: 가장 염려되시는 것이 무엇인지 말씀해 주시겠습니까?

Patient: 예. 심장이 매우 빨리 뛰어요.

Doctor: 알겠습니다. 처음 시작된 때가 언제인가요?

Patient: 지난 화요일부터요.

Doctor: 운동을 할 때 왼쪽 목, 어깨, 팔 또는 가슴에 통증을 느끼나요?

Patient: 제 생각에는 때때로 운동을 한 후 가슴에 통증을 느낍니다.

Doctor: 통증을 설명해 주시겠습니까?

Patient: 예. 가슴 부위를 꽉 조이는 듯한 느낌입니다.

Doctor: 전에도 이런 적이 있었습니까?

Patient: 예. 약 한달 전에도 이러했습니다.

Doctor: 다른 증상도 있나요?

Patient: 예. 어지럼증도 있습니다.

Doctor: 가족 중에 비슷한 증상으로 아픈 사람이 있나요?

Patient: 아니오. 내가 왜 이런 증상이 있는지 알려주시겠습니까?

Doctor: 내 소견에 앞서 먼저 몇 가지 검사를 하겠습니다.

Patient: 별 일 아니었으면 하네요.

5. 나의 증상 설명하기

C. 뻣뻣하고 아픈 무릎관절

Doctor: 몇 가지 고려해볼 사항이 있군요. 무릎부터 먼저 시작하겠습니다. 통증에 대해 설명해 주시겠습니까?

Patient: 무릎관절이 뻣뻣하고 아파요.

Doctor: 처음 통증을 느낀 시기가 언제 인가요?

Patient: 음, 약 이 주 전부터 아프기 시작했어요.

Doctor: 통증이 얼마나 심한가요?

Patient: 아주 심합니다.

Doctor: 하루 중 어느 특정한 때에 통증이 더 악화되나요?

Patient: 예. 통증이 밤에 더 심해집니다. 참을 수가 없을 정도입니다.

Doctor: 통증을 완화시키는 것이 있습니까?

Patient: 아직까지는 없습니다. 진통제도 효과가 없습니다.

Doctor: 음. 혈액검사를 포함한 몇 가지 검사를 하겠습니다. 또한, 무릎 엑스레이도 찍겠습니다.

Patient: 알겠습니다.

5. 나의 증상 설명하기

D. 아픈 눈

Doctor: 어디가 아프십니까?

Patient: 음. 내 생각에 시력이 나빠진 것 같아요. 때때로 내 앞에 있는 것도 잘 안보입니다.

Doctor: 좀 더 자세히 설명해 주시겠습니까?

Patient: 예. 내가 책이나 신문을 읽을 때, 글자가 또렷해 보이지 않아요. 심지어 밝은 불빛이 있는 데도 침침해 보입니다.

Doctor: 시력 검사를 먼저 하겠습니다. 다른 염려 사항이 있습니까?

Patient: 예. 오른쪽 눈에 먼지 같고 작은 벌레 같은 것들이 떠다니는 것 같은 부유물들이 갑자기 더 많아 졌어요. 또한 최근에 제 눈이 빛에 더 민감해진 것 같습니다.

Doctor: 알겠습니다. 안압 검사와 이러한 증상들의 원인을 알기 위해 안압 검사와 몇 가지 눈검사가 필요합니다.

Patient: 심각한가요?

Doctor: 검사 후에 말씀 드리겠습니다.

6. 독해구문
봄철 앨러지

봄은 꽃이 피고 나무들이 새싹을 틔우는 것을 뜻하나, 만일 당신이 봄철 앨러지를 겪는 수백만 명 중 한 사람이라면 봄은 재채기, 코 막힘, 콧물과 그 밖의 고통스러운 증상들을 의미하기도 합니다.

꽃가루 앨러지와 앨러지 비염이라고도 불리는 봄철 앨러지는 당신을 고통스럽게 합니다. 하지만 당신이 조화와 인공잔디로 대신 하기 전에, 봄철 앨러지를 완화하기 위한 몇 가지 간단한 방법들을 시도해 보세요.

앨러지 발생요인에 대한 노출을 줄이세요.

앨러지의 징후와 증상을 발생시키는 많은 요인들(앨러지 유발인자)에 대한 노출을 감소시킬 수 있는 방법들이 많이 있습니다.

건조하고 바람 부는 날에는 실내에 머무르세요 - 가장 좋은 외출시간은 공기 중의 꽃가루가 많이 제거된 비가 흠뻑 온 후입니다.

앨러지 발생요인을 자극시키는 잔디 깎는 일, 잡초 뽑는 일과 그 밖의 정원 일을 다른 사람에게 위임하세요.

외출 시 입었던 옷을 갈아입으세요. 그리고 당신의 피부와 머리카락에 묻은 꽃가루를 샤워를 해서 씻어내세요.

빨래를 밖에 널지 마세요 - 꽃가루가 이불보와 수건에 달라붙을 수 있습니다.

바깥 일을 할 때 마스크를 착용하세요.

Chapter 4

꽃가루의 수치(=화분계측)가 높아질 때 추가적인 대비책을 마련하세요.

계절 앨러지의 징후와 증상은 공기 중 꽃가루가 많이 있을 때 악화될 수 있습니다. 다음의 방법들이 노출의 감소에 도움이 될 수 있습니다.

꽃가루 수치와 현재의 꽃가루 양을 지역방송과 라디오, 신문 또는 인터넷을 통해 확인하세요.

만일 꽃가루의 수치가 높다는 방송이 방영 된다면, 증상이 시작되기 전에 앨러지 약을 드세요.

밤이나 꽃가루 수치가 높은 시간대에 문과 창문을 닫으세요.

꽃가루 수치가 가장 높은 이른 아침에 외부 활동을 피하세요.

Chapter 5
Pain
통증

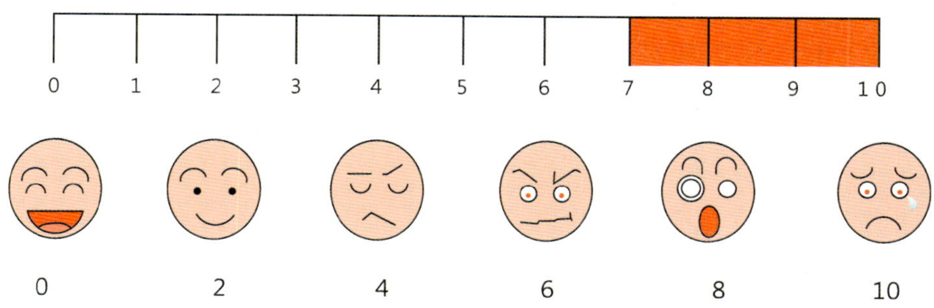

1. Character of Pain
통증의 성질(종류)

- **Key Words, 주요어휘**

  A. 몹시 괴로운 통증
  B. 날카롭게 아픈 통증
  Quiz: 내 단어장 점검하기
  C. 쪼는 듯한 통증
  D. 타는 듯한 통증
  E. 근육통이 있는, 몸이 쑤시는
  Quiz: 내 단어장 점검하기
  F. 피부가 벗겨져(까져서) 쓰라린
  G. 만졌을 때 또는 촉진 시 느끼는 통증
  H. 꽉 조여오는 통증
  I. 콕콕 찌르는 듯한 통증
  J. 묵직하게 지속적으로 아픈 통증
  K. 방사통
  L. 저릿저릿한 감각
  M. 지끈거리는/욱신거리는 통증
  Quiz: 내 단어장 점검하기
  - Drill: Word Search Puzzle, 연습문제: 단어퍼즐

- **Key Expressions, 주요구문: 어떻게 아프세요?**
  - Words, 어휘
  - Drill, 연습문제

- **Word Review, 어휘복습**

Key Words

A. 몹시 괴로운 통증

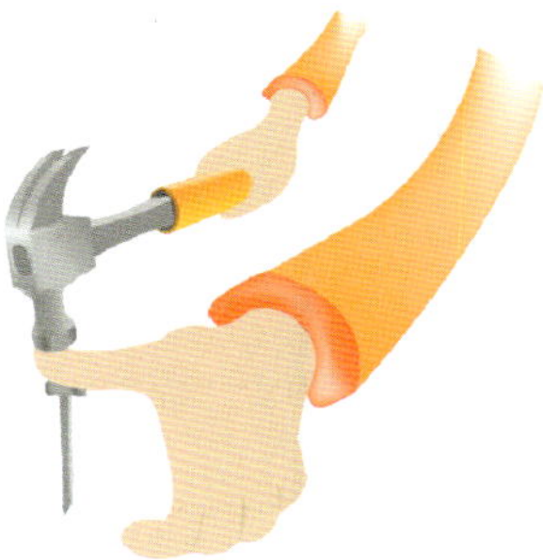

Splitting pain: 쪼개질 듯한 통증

Tearing or ripping pain: 찢어지는 듯한 통증

Excruciating pain: 참을 수 없을 만큼 아픈 통증

Terrible pain: 끔찍한 통증

Colic pain (It is severe pain in your stomach and bowels)**:** 산통-위, 장에 나타나는 극심한 통증

B. 날카롭게 아픈 통증

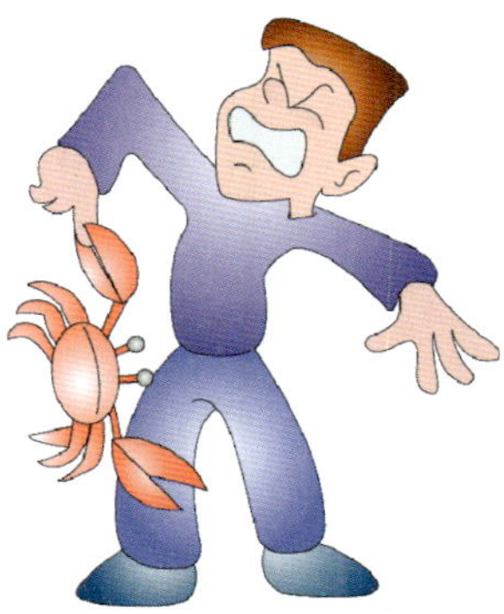

Stabbing pain: 칼로 찌르는 듯한 통증

Sharp pain: 날카롭게 느껴지는 통증

Twinge pain/Smart pain (A sudden short sharp pain)**:** 예리한 급성 통증

Shooting pain: 쏘는 듯한 통증

Lancinating pain/Piercing pain: 찌르는 듯한 극심한 통증

QUIZ: 내 단어장 점검하기 !!

아래 단어 및 문장을 읽고 알맞은 통증의 이름을 적어보세요.

A sudden short sharp pain: ....

Splitting pain: ....

Smart pain: ....

Excruciating pain: ....

Twinge pain: ....

Colic pain: ....

Sharp pain: ....

Shooting pain: ....

Lancinating pain: ....

Terrible pain: ....

Tearing or ripping pain: ....

Stabbing pain: ....

Piercing pain: ....

It is severe pain in your stomach and bowels: ....

....

C. 쪼는 듯한 통증

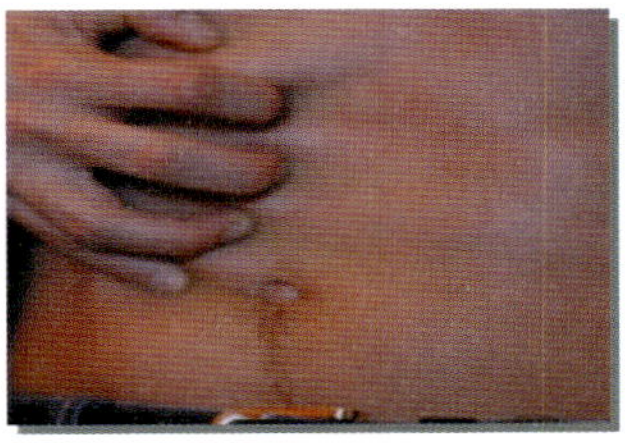

Gnawing pain: 쪼는 듯한 통증

It is burning or gnawing feeling in the stomach area lasting 30 minutes to 3 hours; commonly accompanies ulcers.

D. 타는 듯한 통증

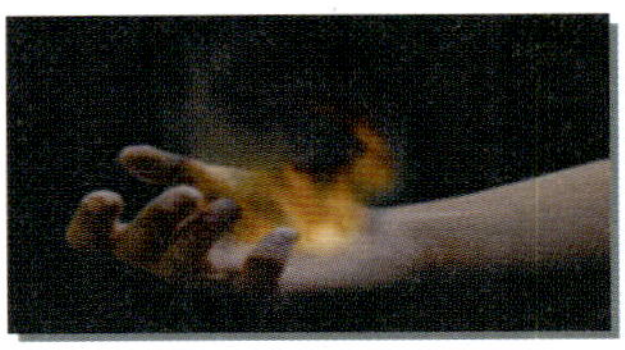

Burning pain/Burning sensation: 작열통/작열감

It feels as if a part of your body is touching something hot.

E. 근육통이 있는, 몸이 쑤시는

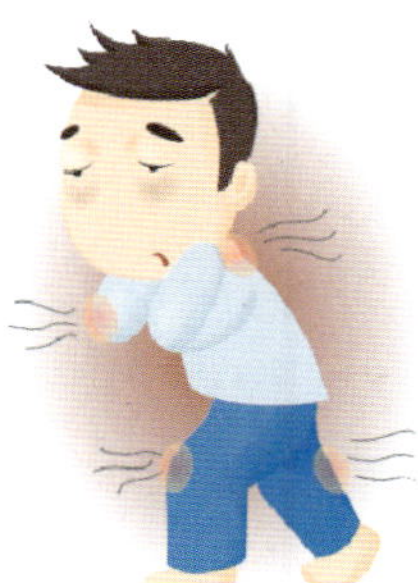

Sore: 근육통이 있는, 몸이 쑤시는

Soreness: 통증

(Muscle) Soreness: 근육통(심한 운동 후에 느끼는)

My arms are sore.

My leg muscles are very sore after the marathon.

QUIZ: 내 단어장 점검하기 !!

아래 단어 및 문장을 읽고 알맞은 통증의 이름을 적어보세요.

Sore: ....

Gnawing pain: ....

Burning pain: ....

Muscle soreness: ....

Burning sensation: ....

My arms are sore: ....

Soreness: ....

My leg muscles are very sore after the marathon: ....

....

It feels as if a part of your body is touching something hot: ....

F. 피부가 벗겨져(까져서) 쓰라린

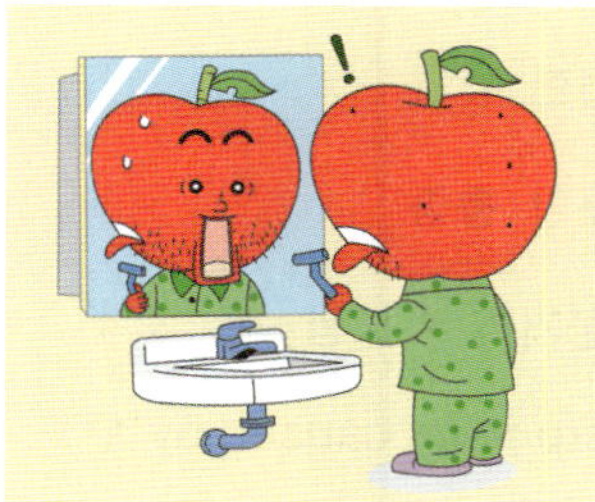

Raw (feeling): 쓰라린

There were raw patches on her feet where the shoes had rubbed.

I have a raw sensation in my gums and in my soft palate.

G. 만졌을 때 또는 촉진 시 느끼는 통증

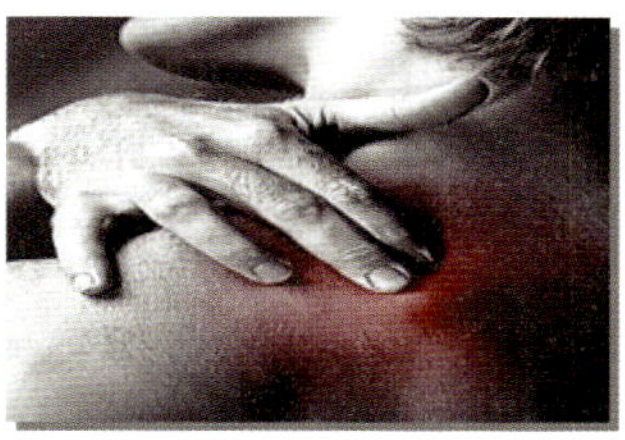

Tenderness: 눌렀을 때 느끼는 통증

It is pain or discomfort when an affected area is touched.

H. 꽉 조여오는 통증

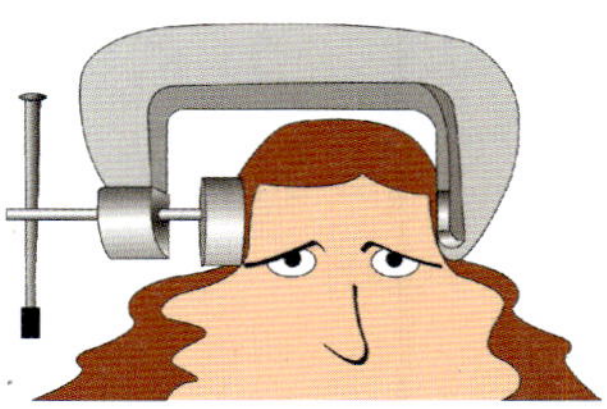

Pressing pain: 누르는 듯한 통증

Squeezing pain: 조이는 듯한 통증

Constricting pain: 꽉 조여오는 듯한 통증

I. 콕콕 찌르는 듯한 통증

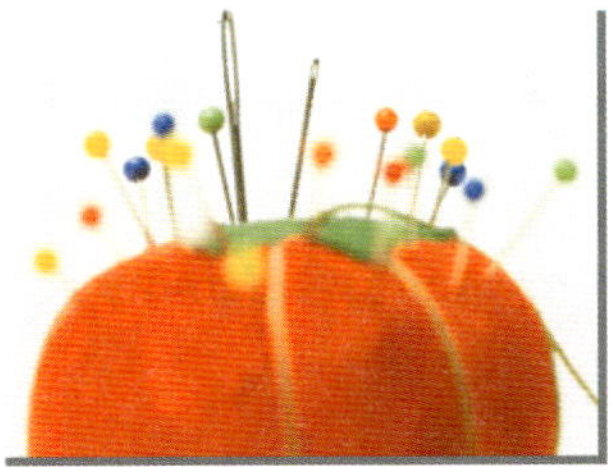

Prickling pain: 찌르는 듯한 통증

Pinching pain: 꼬집는 듯한 통증

Stinging sensation: 따끔거리는 느낌

It is a quick feeling of sharp pain, caused by a sharp object making a hole on your skin.

J. 묵직하게 지속적으로 아픈 통증

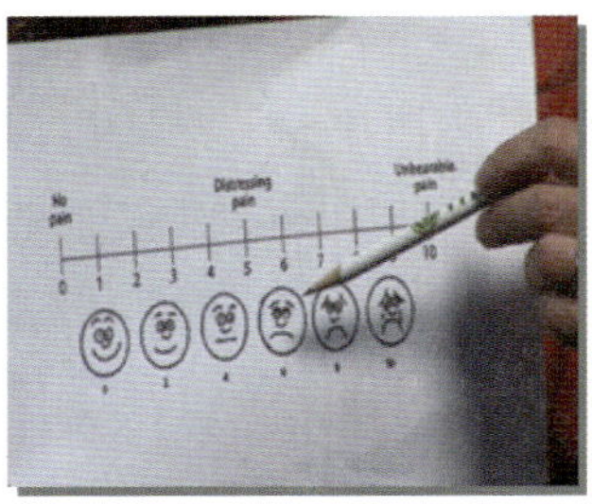

Dull pain: 둔통

It is not very strong but continues for a long time.

Ache or Aching: 묵직하며 지속되는 통증

It is continuous and unpleasant, but usually not very strong pain.

K. 방사통

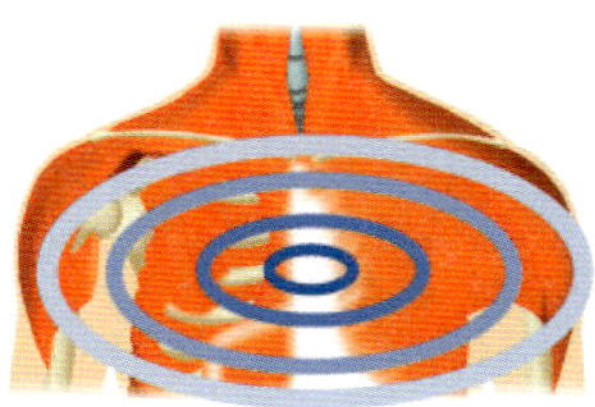

Radiation pain: 방사통

It is a pain that moves from the original area outwards to other parts of the body.

L. 저릿저릿한 감각

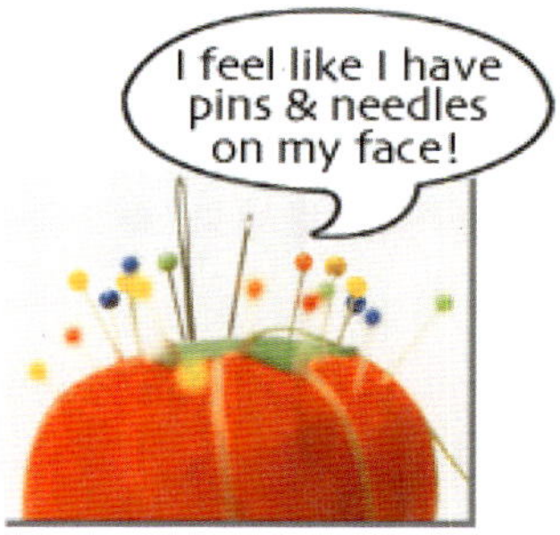

Tingling sensation: 저릿저릿한 감각

Pins and needles: 저린 느낌

I have pins and needles in my feet.

M. 지끈거리는/욱신거리는 통증

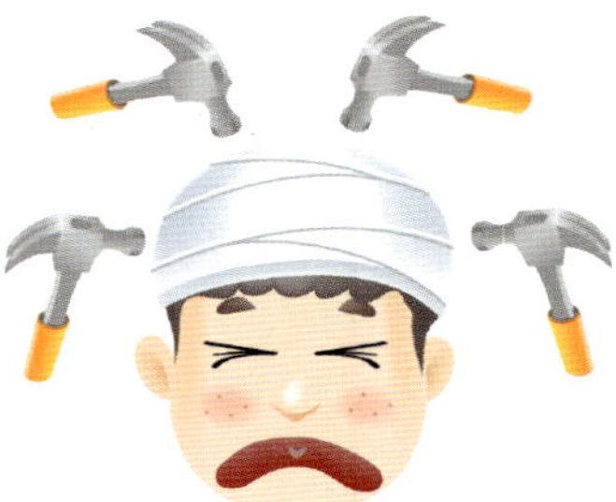

Pounding (pain): 지끈거리는 (통증)

Pounding headache: 지끈거리는 두통

Throbbing pain: 욱신거리는 통증

QUIZ: 내 단어장 점검하기 !!

아래 단어 및 문장을 읽고 알맞은 통증의 이름을 적어보세요.

Pressing pain: ....

Raw (feeling): ....

Constricting pain: ....

Tenderness: ....

Squeezing pain: ....

Dull pain: ....

Prickling pain: ....

Radiation pain: ....

Pinching pain: ....

Ache or Aching: ....

Stinging sensation: ....

Throbbing pain: ....

Tingling sensation: ....

Pounding (pain): ....

Pounding headache: ....

Pins and needles: ....

It is pain or discomfort when an affected area is touched:

....

It is not very strong but continues for a long time: ....

....

It is a quick feeling of sharp pain, caused by a sharp object making a hole on your skin: ....

It is continuous and unpleasant, but usually not very strong pain: ....

It is a pain that moves from the original area outwards to other parts of the body: ....

Drill: 아래의 단어를 Word Search Puzzle에서 찾아보세요.

J	O	M	R	B	T	S	F	I	Q	T	U	R	S	T	V	N	S
E	F	M	A	S	B	R	D	V	Y	W	M	V	Y	D	O	T	P
X	J	T	D	O	U	P	Y	G	M	I	C	R	P	O	I	V	A
C	O	N	I	R	R	Q	J	K	U	T	Q	I	E	N	M	U	B
R	N	C	A	E	N	Q	G	V	H	J	T	I	G	T	P	H	O
U	A	W	T	N	I	T	M	T	Q	F	E	I	E	A	U	C	P
C	Q	B	I	E	N	G	L	P	A	X	N	W	A	E	H	O	M
I	L	S	O	S	G	N	R	K	O	G	D	W	Q	N	Q	S	N
A	P	I	N	S		A	N	D		N	E	E	D	L	E	S	Q
T	U	R		N	S	W	V	S	M	A	R	T		P	A	I	N
I	X	R	P	F	E	I	E	C	B	K	N	H	X	L	G	N	W
N	B	I	A	R	N	N	F	A	N	N	E	R	G	S	H	W	C
G	J	H	I	W	S	G	S	B	V	O	S	O	L	G	R	R	C
	D	H	N	A	A		I	Y	R	G	S	B	B	P	E	F	V
P	I	T	T	J	T	P	Q	X	Q	G	R	B	B	J	N	M	H
A	Y	I	G	L	I	A	C	A	D	K	P	I	H	Q	U	V	C
I	O	R	A	C	O	I	Y	R	K	L	E	N	R	W	E	W	V
N	C	Y	G	A	N	N	U	Q	W	S	N	G	J	R	P	O	Q

참을 수 없을 만큼 아픈 통증, 예리한 급성 통증, 쪼는 듯한 통증, 작열감, 통증, 쓰라린, 눌렀을 때 느끼는 통증, 따끔거리는 느낌, 방사통, 저린 느낌, 욱신거리는 통증

Key Expressions

어떻게 아프세요?

Q1. Can you describe the pain please?

A1. It's like a heavy weight pressing on my chest.

Q2. What's the pain like?

A2. It's like a burning pain.

Q3. What is the character of the pain?

A3. It's very sharp and stabbing.

Words

heavy weight: 무거운 것

character of pain: 통증의 성질(어떠한 통증)

burning pain: 타는 듯한 통증

sharp: 날카롭게 느껴지는 통증

stabbing: 칼로 찌르는 듯한 통증

Drill: Q1-Q6을 영작하세요.

정답은 전 페이지의 Key Expressions을 참고하세요

Q1. 통증을 설명해 주시겠습니까?

____

Q2. 통증이 어떠한가요?

____

Q3. 어떠한 통증인가요?

____

Q4. 무거운 것이 제 가슴을 누르는 듯 합니다.

____

Q5. 타는 듯한 통증입니다.

____

Q6. 칼로 찌르는 듯이 예리한 통증입니다.

____

Word Review: 위의 단어들을 복습하는 공간입니다. 정답은 Key Words를 참고하세요.

뜻: In English

쪼개질 듯한 통증:______________________

찢어지는 듯한 통증:______________________

참을 수 없을 만큼 아픈 통증:______________________

끔찍한 통증:______________________

산통-위, 장에 나타나는 극심한 통증:______________________

칼로 찌르는 듯한 통증:______________________

날카롭게 느껴지는 통증:______________________

예리한 급성 통증:______________________

쏘는 듯한 통증:______________________

찌르는 듯한 극심한 통증:______________________

쪼는 듯한 통증:______________________

작열통/작열감:______________________

근육통이 있는, 몸이 쑤시는:______________________

근육통:______________________

쓰라린:____________________

눌렀을 때 느끼는 통증:____________________

누르는 듯한 통:____________________

조이는 듯한 통증:____________________

꽉 조여오는 듯한 통증:____________________

찌르는 듯한 통증:____________________

꼬집는 듯한 통증:____________________

따끔거리는 느낌:____________________

둔통:____________________

묵직하며 지속되는 통증:____________________

방사통:____________________

저릿저릿한 감각:____________________

저린 느낌:____________________

지끈거리는 (통증):____________________

지끈거리는 두통:____________________

욱신거리는 통증:____________________

통증:____________________

2. Locations of Pain
통증부위

- **Key Words, 주요어휘**
  - Quiz: 내 단어장 점검하기
- **Key Expressions, 주요구문: 어느 부위가 아프세요?**
  - Drill, 연습문제
- **Describing My Pain: Pain in the Neck, 나의 통증 설명하기, 목의 통증**
  - Dialogue, 대화
  - Words, 어휘
  - Review, 복습
- **Word Review, 어휘복습**

Key Words

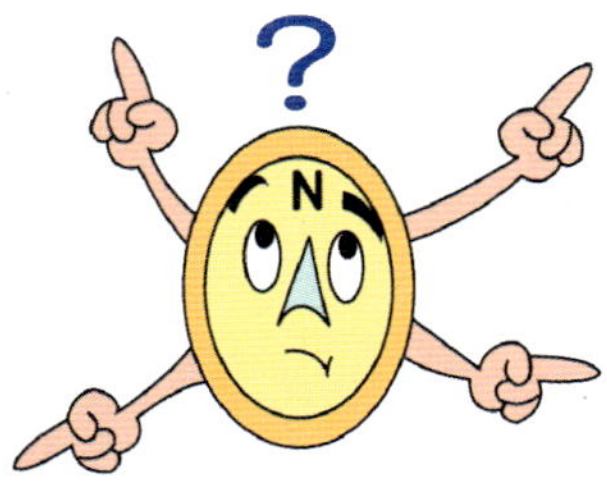

Head: 두부	Back: 등	Extremities (Arms/Legs): 사지(팔/다리)
Front part of the head: 전면/머리 앞부분	Upper back: 상부/허리 윗부위	Arms
Top of the head: 정수리 부위	Lower back: 하부/허리부위	Upper arm: 상완
Back of the head: 후면/머리 뒷부분		Lower arm (=forearm): 전완
Left-side of the head: 좌측/머리 왼쪽		Legs
Right-side of the head: 우측/머리 오른쪽		Upper leg (=Thigh): 상부(허벅지)
		Lower leg: 하부 (=Calf): 종아리

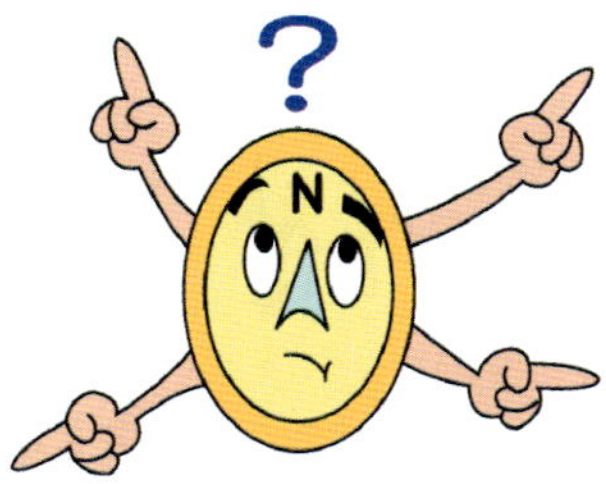

Abdomen (Belly): 복부	Radiation: 전이	Superficial/ Deep/No specific area: 표면/심부/비특정
Right Upper Quadrant (RUQ, 우상부) Right upper side of my belly: 배의 오른 쪽 윗 부위 **Right Lower Quadrant (RLQ, 우하부)** Right lower side of my belly: 배의 오른 쪽 아랫 부위 **Left Upper Quadrant (LUQ, 좌상부)** Left upper side of my belly: 배의 왼 쪽 윗 부위. **Left Lower Quadrant (LLQ , 좌하부)** Left lower side of my belly: 배의 왼 쪽 아랫 부위.	**Moving from one area to another:** 통증이 다른 부위로 옮겨가는	**Close to the surface:** 겉에서 느껴지는 통증 **Deep inside:** 속에서 느껴지는 통증 **All over:** 몸 전체

QUIZ: 내 단어장 점검하기 !!

아래 단어 및 문장을 읽고 알맞은 통증의 이름을 적어보세요.

Front part of the head: ....

Top of the head: ....

Back of the head: ....

Left-side of the head: ....

Right-side of the head: ....

Upper back: ....

Deep inside: ....

Lower back: ....

Forearm: ....

Right upper side of my belly: ....

Left upper side of my belly: ....

Right lower side of my belly: ....

Left lower side of my belly: ....

All over: ....

Moving from one area to another: ....

No specific area: ....

Radiation: ....

Superficial: ....

Upper arm: ....

Upper leg/Lower leg: ....

Thigh: ....

Key Expressions

어느 부위가 아프세요?

Q1. Where is your pain located?

A1. I have a bad pain in the upper right side of my stomach since last night.

Q2. Does the pain radiate anywhere?/Does it start in one place and spread to another?

A2. Yes, it does. It starts from my neck and moves to my left arm.

Q3. Is the pain deep inside or close to the surface?

A3. It feels like it's inside, and not on the surface.

Q4. Does it hurt in one part of your body or more than one place?

A4. I have severe pain all over my body without any reason.

Q5. Is the pain on one side only or on both sides?

A5. This weird pain is only on one side of my jaw.

Q6. Where is your pain concentrated?

A6. I have pain in my right upper thigh.

Drill: Q1-Q12를 영작하세요.

정답은 전 페이지의 Key Expressions을 참고하세요

Q1. 어느 부위가 아프세요?

____

Q2. 통증이 한 곳에서 시작되어 다른 곳으로 퍼지나요?

____

Q3. 속이 아픈가요 아니면 겉에서 통증을 느끼나요?

____

Q4. 몸의 한 부위가 아픈가요, 아니면 여러 곳이 아픈가요?

____

Q5. 한쪽 부위만 아픈가요 또는 양쪽 부위 다 아픈가요?

____

Q6. 어디가 가장 아프세요?

____

Q7. 겉이 아니고 속에서 아픈 것 같아요.

____

Q8. 이유 없이 온몸이 심하게 아파요.

____

Q9. 지난 밤부터 배의 오른쪽 위 부위가 심하게 아파요.

____

Q10. 이상한 통증이 턱의 한 쪽 부위에서만 느껴져요.

____

Q11. 통증이 목에서 시작해서 왼쪽 팔로 옮겨 가요.

____

Q12. 허벅지의 오른쪽 윗 부분에 통증이 느껴져요.

____

Describing My Pain

Pain in the Neck

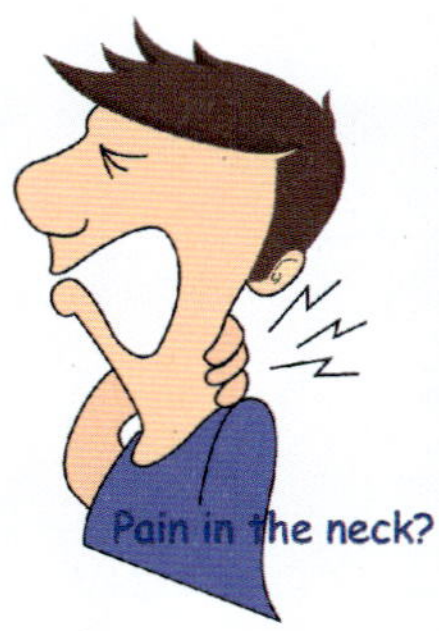

Doctor: What brings you here, sir?

Patient: Well, I work in front of the computer 8 to 10 hours per day on average, and I have noticed the pain in my neck nowadays.

Doctor: Can you describe your pain, please?

Patient: It feels stiff.

Doctor: Does the pain come and go or do you have it all the time?

Patient: It's on and off.

Doctor: Does the pain move to some other areas?

Patient: Yes. It moves to my shoulder and right upper arm.

Doctor: Do you have tingling or numbness in your wrists and hands?

Patient: Yes. I have pins and needles in my right wrist and hand.

Doctor: Did you ever have this episode before?

Patient: No, I didn't.

Doctor: I see. I am going to examine the alignment of your neck to make sure they are working normally. Also, I will check your neck for flexibility. Please follow my instructions.

Patient: Okay.

Words

stiff: 뻣뻣한

upper arm: 상완

forearm: 전완

tingling: 저릿저릿한

numbness: 무감각한

pins and needles: 저린 느낌

Review: 각각의 구문을 영작하세요.
정답은 전 페이지의 Dialogue를 참고하세요.

Doctor: 어디가 아프셔서 오셨어요?

Patient: Well, I work in front of the computer 8 to 10 hours per day on average, and I have noticed the pain in my neck nowadays.

Doctor: 통증을 설명해 주시겠습니까?

Patient: It feels stiff.

Doctor: 통증은 간헐적인가요 아니면 항상 아픈가요?

Patient: It's on and off.

Doctor: 통증이 다른 곳으로도 퍼지나요?

Patient: Yes. It moves to my shoulder and right upper arm.

Doctor: 손목과 손에 저리거나 감각이 무뎌지는 것을 느끼십니까?

Patient: Yes. I have pins and needles in my right wrist and hand.

Doctor: 전에도 이런 적이 있었나요?

Patient: No I didn't.

Doctor: 알겠습니다. 제가 환자분의 목이 정상적인 선열을 가지고 있는지 검사하겠습니다.

또한 유연성도 확인하겠습니다.

제 지시사항을 따라주세요.

Patient: Okay.

Word Review: 위의 단어들을 복습하는 공간입니다.
정답은 Key Words를 참고하세요.

뜻: In English

통증의 전이 :______________________________

우측/머리 오른쪽:______________________________

전면/머리 앞부분:______________________________

정수리 부위:______________________________

후면/머리 뒷부분:______________________________

겉에서 느껴지는 통증:______________________________

몸 전체:______________________________

허리부위/허리 윗 부위:______________________________

상완:______________________________

배의 오른 쪽 윗 부위:______________________________

배의 오른 쪽 아랫 부위:______________________________

배의 왼 쪽 윗 부위:______________________________

배의 왼 쪽 아랫 부위:______________________________

비특정: ______________________________

통증이 다른 부위로 옮겨가는: ______________________________

속에서 느껴지는 통증: ______________________________

전완: ______________________________

3. Story of My Pain
나의 통증 이야기

- **Reading Material, 독해구문**

A. Burning sensation, 작열감

- Words, 어휘

B. Pressing pain on lower back, 허리에 있는 눌리는 듯한 통증

- Words, 어휘

C. Gums are white with raw and painful feeling, 잇몸이 창백하며 쓰라리고 아픕니다.

- Words, 어휘

Reading Material

A. Burning Sensation

A burning sensation, either in a particular area of the body or over a wide range throughout, is not a pleasant thing.

It can also be an indication of a number of underlying problems.

Depending on other symptoms that accompany the burning sensation, the cause could be anything from a reaction to severe trauma to an indication of vascular disease.

Words

a wide range throughout: 전체에 걸친

a number of: 많은

indication: 징후

underlying problems: 기저질환들

accompany: 동반하다

severe trauma: 심각한 외상

vascular disease: 혈관 질환

B. Pressing pain on lower back

I am on antibiotics currently for a sinus infection, and I have had this pressing pain in the right side of my lower back. Should I go to the doc to see if it's a kidney infection? The pain comes and goes and it's never really severe. I have no other symptoms of a kidney infection. However, I cannot lay on my right side because of the pain, and sometimes I feel it in the left side, but always in my lower back.

Thanks so much for your advice!

Words

antibiotics: 항생제

I am on antibiotics.: 나는 항생제를 복용 중입니다.

sinus infection: 부비동염

lower back: 허리

doc: doctor의 격식을 차리지 않은 표현

pressing pain: 누르는 듯한 통증

kidney infection: 신장염

lay on my right side: 오른쪽으로 눕다

C. Gums are white with raw and painful feeling.

I recently went to the dentist to have a tooth filled. He filled the tooth, but after that the tooth became very painful and my gums began to turn white with painful and raw feeling. After that, I later went back and had the tooth extracted, and my gums are still very white looking with painful and raw feeling. It has been over 3 weeks since the extraction and the hole that the tooth was in is nearly healed up. My question is why my gums are in this condition. My husband has had several tooth extractions and he had never experienced anything like this. It's been over 6 weeks since it began.

Words

to have a tooth filled: 충치치료를 위해

gums: 잇몸

raw feeling: 쓰라린

have the tooth extracted: 이를 발치했다

nearly healed up: 거의 치유가 되었다

extraction: 발치

4. The Concept of the Pain
통증의 개념

- **PAIN** (noun)
- **PAINFUL** (adjective)
- **ACHE** (noun)
- **ACHE** (verb)
- **PAINS and ACHES** (noun)
- **SORE** (noun)
- **SORENESS** (noun)
- **SORE** (adjective)
- **HURT** (verb)
- **Drill: Fill in the blanks, 연습문제**

PAIN (noun)

- the feeling you have when part of your body hurts

She is in pain.

My pain intensifies.

I didn't take any pain medication, so the pain increased.

The pain grows stronger.

I am suffering from chronic back pain.

Pain wears off.

Pain stops.

Pain disappears.

PAINFUL (adjective**)**

- that causes pain (can be both physical and emotional)

Emotionally:

It is still painful for her to talk about the loss of her father.

Physically:

He was complaining of his painful and swollen knee joints.

ACHE (noun)

- pain that lasts for a long time

I have a headache.

I have a stomachache.

She has a toothache.

He has a heartache.

ACHE (verb)

- to feel a continuous pain

I ached all over.

My back ached badly.

My feet really ached.

PAINS and ACHES (noun)

- many small pains which he/she feels simultaneously, but no real health problems

Many old people suffered from all kinds of **pains and aches.**

SORE (noun)

- a painful, often red spot on your body caused by a wound or infection

The patient developed a bedsore.

I have bad cold sores on my lips.

SORENESS (noun)

- A pain or irritation

Muscle soreness is most frequently felt when you begin a new exercise program, change your exercise routine, or dramatically increase the duration or intensity of your exercise routine.

SORE (adjective)

- painful as a result of a wound, infection or too much exercise

I have a sore throat.

Both of my feet are sore.

HURT (verb)

- can mean not only physical pain but also emotional pain as well

to feel pain

to cause pain in a part of your body

Emotionally:

Your remarks hurt me deeply.

I didn't mean to hurt you.

Physically:

My ankle still hurts quite badly.

I have to sit down because my legs are hurting me badly.

She fell and hurt her leg slightly.

My knees hurt when I run.

Drill: 알맞은 어휘를 넣어 문장을 완성하세요.

Fill in the blanks choosing the best word: *pain, painful, ache, hurt or sore?*

1. A bee sting can be extremely ______________.
2. She has a chest ________________.
3. She completed the marathon and her body _____ all over.
4. He made an appointment with the dentist because he couldn't put up with his ______________ any longer.
5. I have an ear____________.
6. I was badly ____________ in the accident.
7. She is suffering from chronic back_________.
8. Gardening aggravates my ____________.
9. That spot is very _____________, doctor.
10. After I took the analgesic, the ____________ wore off.
11. I can't walk. My ankle ______________.
12. My grandmother usually suffers from a lot of __________ and __________.
13. I am very ______________ because of all that exercise.
14. Despite all the chiropractic adjustments, my back still ________ me.
15. He has a _________throat.

5. Timing of Pain
통증발생 시간

- **Key Words, 주요어휘**
  - ■ Quiz: 내 단어장 점검하기
- **Key Expressions, 주요구문**

통증이 언제부터 시작되었나요?

- ◆ Words, 어휘
- ◆ Drill, 연습문제

통증이 하루 중 특정한 시간대에 발생하나요?

- ◆ Words, 어휘
- ◆ Drill, 연습문제

아프신지 얼마나 되셨습니까?

- ◆ Words, 어휘
- ◆ Drill, 연습문제

예전에도 이런 통증이 있었나요?

- ◆ Words, 어휘
- ◆ Drill, 연습문제

- **Describing My Pain: Painful Knee Joints, 나의 통증 설명하기: 무릎관절통증**
  - ■ Dialogue, 대화
  - ■ Words, 어휘
  - ■ Review, 복습
- **Word Review, 어휘복습**

Key Words

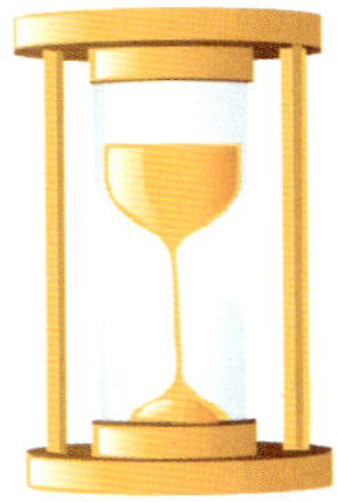

Time of Day: 하루 중 특정한 시간	Several ~: ~일/~주/~달	For ~: ~동안	Since ~: ~부터
Early morning (midnight-5am): 새벽 Morning (5am-9am): 이른 아침 Late morning (9am-noon): 늦은 아침	Several days: 며칠	For about half an hour: 대략 30분 정도	Since last night: 지난밤부터
Early afternoon (noon-3pm): 이른 오후 Late afternoon (3pm-6pm): 늦은 오후	Several weeks: 몇 주	For about five days: 약 5일 정도 For a couple of days: 2~3일 동안	Since several days ago: 며칠 전부터
Evening (6pm-9pm): 저녁 Night (9pm-midnight): 밤	Several months: 몇 달	For a week: 일주일 동안 For a fortnight: 2주 동안	Since more than a week ago: 일주일도 더 되었음 Since a month ago: 한달 전부터
All day and night: 하루 종일			Since right before coming to Korea: 한국에 오기 바로 전부터

QUIZ: 내 단어장 점검하기 !!

아래의 표에 알맞은 단어 및 구문을 적으세요.

Time of Day: 하루 중 특정한 시간	Several ~: ~일/~주/~달	For ~: ~동안	Since ~: ~부터
Early morning (midnight-5am):	Several days:	For about half an hour:	Since last night:
Morning (5am-9am):	Several weeks:	For about five days:	Since several days ago:
Late morning (9am-noon):	Several months:	For a couple of days:	Since more than a week ago:
Early afternoon (noon-3pm):		For a week:	Since a month ago:
Late afternoon (3pm-6pm):		For a fortnight:	Since right before coming to Korea:
Evening (6pm-9pm):			
Night (9pm-midnight):			
All day and night:			

Key Expressions

통증이 언제부터 시작되었나요?

Q1. When did the pain start?

A1. It started since last night.

Q2. When did your headaches begin?

A2. They began about a week ago.

Q3. When did you first notice the pain?

A3. I noticed it a couple of days ago.

Words

since last night: 지난밤부터

a week ago: 일 주일 전

a couple of days ago: 2~3일 전

Drill: Q1-Q6을 영작하세요.

정답은 전 페이지의 Key Expressions을 참고하세요.

Q1. 통증이 언제부터 시작되었지요?

____

Q2. 두통이 언제부터 시작되었나요?

____

Q3. 통증이 언제 처음 시작되었나요?

____

Q4. 약 일 주 전부터 시작되었어요.

____

Q5. 약 2~3일 전에 알게 되었어요.

____

Q6. 어제 밤부터 시작되었습니다.

____

Key Expressions

통증이 하루 중 특정한 시간대에 발생하나요?

Q1. Does your pain begin during the day or at night?

A1. I think my pain begins during the day time.

Q2. Do your headaches come on at any particular time of the day?

A2. I think they seem to come on early in the morning. I notice them when I wake up.

Q3. Is your pain there all the time or does it come on at any particular time?

A3. Well, I am fine during the day time, but I wake up at night because of the pain.

Words

during the day time: 낮 시간 동안에

at any particular time of the day: 하루 중 특정한 시간대에

early in the morning: 이른 아침

Drill: Q1-Q8을 영작하세요.

정답은 전 페이지의 Key Expressions를 참고하세요.

Q1. 통증이 낮에 시작되나요 또는 밤에 시작되나요?

____

Q2. 두통이 하루 중 특정한 시간대에 시작되나요?

____

Q3. 항상 통증을 느끼나요 아니면 특정 시간에 통증을 느끼나요?

____

Q4. 제 생각에 통증이 낮에 시작되는 것 같아요.

____

Q5. 제 생각에는 두통이 이른 아침에 시작되는 것 같습니다.

____

Q6. 아침에 일어날 때 통증을 느낍니다.

____

Q7. 낮에는 괜찮습니다.

____

Q8. 밤에는 통증 때문에 자다가 깨어납니다.

____

Key Expressions

아프신지 얼마나 되셨습니까?

Q1. How long have you had your chest pain?

A1. I have been having this chest pain for about two months now.

Q2. How long has the toothache been bothering you?

A2. It's been bothering me since last week.

Q3. How long have you been suffering from your lower back pain?

A3. This episode of lower back pain has lasted for longer than 4 weeks.

Q4. How long have you had the canker sores?

A4. Two or three days.

Words

lumbago/lower back pain: 요통

apthous ulcer/canker sores: 구내염

this episode of ~: 이번에 발생한 ~질병

Drill: Q1-Q8을 영작하세요.

정답은 전 페이지의 Key Expressions을 참고하세요.

Q1. 얼마나 오랫동안 흉통이 있었나요?

____

Q2. 이가 얼마 동안 아프셨나요?

____

Q3. 요통으로 고생 하신지 얼마나 되셨나요?

____

Q4. 구내염이 생긴지 얼마나 되셨나요?

____

Q5. 흉통이 생긴지 약 2개월 되었습니다.

____

Q6. 지난주부터 아팠어요.

____

Q7. 이번에 생긴 허리 통증은 4주 이상 지속되고 있습니다.

____

Q8. 2-3일 정도요.

____

Key Expressions

예전에도 이런 통증이 있었나요?

Q1. Have you had a pain like this before?

A1. No. I have never had a pain like this before. This is a pretty new type of pain to me.

Q2. Have you had lower back pain before?

A2. Yes. I have had lower back pain before, but this episode is different and feels worse.

Q3. If you had the chest pain before, is this pain similar or different?

A3. Well, the pain I have now is quite similar to the one I had last summer.

Words

lower back pain/lumbago: 요통

this episode: 이번에 발생한 통증

chest pain: 흉통

Drill: Q1-Q7을 영작하세요.

정답은 전 페이지의 Key Expression를 참고하세요.

Q1. 전에도 이런 통증을 느끼셨나요?

____

Q2. 이전에도 요통이 있었나요?

____

Q3. 전에도 흉통이 있었다면, 이번 통증은 전과 유사한가요 아니면 다른가요?

____

Q4. 전에 이런 종류의 통증을 느낀 적이 없습니다.

____

Q5. 전에도 요통이 있었지만, 이번 경우는 다르고 통증도 더 심합니다.

____

Q6. 지난 여름에 느꼈던 흉통과 아주 흡사해요.

____

Q7. 내게 새로운 종류의 통증입니다.

____

Describing My Pain

Painful Knee Joints

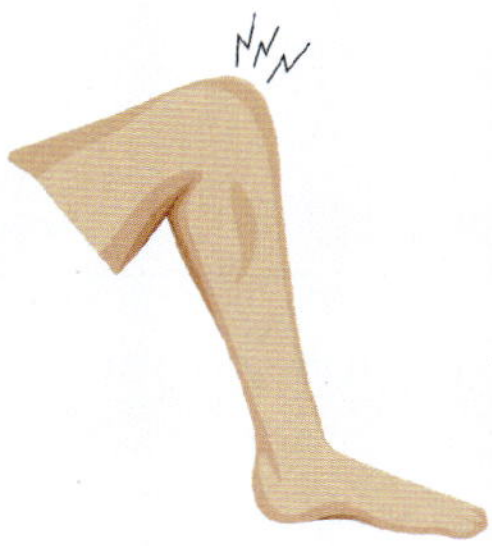

Patient: My knee joints are so painful.

Doctor: When did you first notice your pain?

Patient: I noticed it two days ago when I was climbing the stairs.

Doctor: Is there anything you can do to relieve the pain?

Patient: Well, I think my pain can be relieved by elevation of affected area.

Doctor: How long does it take for the pain to go away?

Patient: It usually takes about a day.

Doctor: I am going to examine your knee, so would you get on the bed and lie on your back, please?

Patient: Alright.

Doctor: Now, I am going to bend your knee. How does that feel?

Patient: Oh, that hurts a lot.

Words

knee joint: 무릎관절

climbing the stairs: 계단을 오르는

elevation of affected area: 아픈 부위를 높이 올림

about=around=approximately: 약, 대략

lie on your back: 등을 대고 눕다

bend your knee: 무릎을 굽히다

Review: 각각의 구문을 영작하세요.

정답은 전 페이지의 Dialogue를 참고하세요.

Patient: My knee joints are so painful.

Doctor: 통증을 처음 느낀 게 언제입니까?

Patient: I noticed it two days ago when I was climbing the stairs.

Doctor: 통증을 경감시키기 위해 하실 수 있는 일이 있습니까?

Patient: Well, I think my pain can be relieved by elevation of affected area.

Doctor: 통증이 사라지는데 얼마나 걸리나요?

Patient: It usually takes about a day.

Doctor: 무릎을 검사하겠으니 침대에 올라오셔서 등을 대고 누우시겠습니까?

Patient: Alright.

Doctor: 무릎을 굽히겠습니다. 느낌이 어떤가요?

Patient: Oh, that hurts a lot.

Word Review: 위의 단어들을 복습하는 공간입니다.
정답은 Key Words를 참고하세요.

뜻: In English

하루 중 특정한 시간: ______________________________

새벽/이른 아침/늦은 아침: ______________________________

2주 동안: ______________________________

약 5일 정도: ______________________________

2~3일 동안: ______________________________

대략 30분 정도: ______________________________

지난밤부터/며칠 전부터: ______________________________

한달 전부터: ______________________________

한국에 오기 바로 전부터: ______________________________

일주일도 더 되었음: ______________________________

몇 주/몇 달/며칠: ______________________________

하루 종일: ______________________________

밤/저녁: ______________________________

이른 오후/늦은 오후: ______________________________

6. Intensity of pain
통증의 강도

- **Key Words, 주요어휘**
  - QUIZ: 내 단어장 점검하기
- **Key Expressions, 주요구문: 통증이 얼마나 심한가요?**
  - Words, 어휘
  - Drill, 연습문제
- **Describing My Pain: Chest Pain, 나의 통증 설명하기: 흉통**
  - Dialogue, 대화
  - Words, 어휘
  - Review, 복습
- **Word Review, 어휘복습**

Key Words

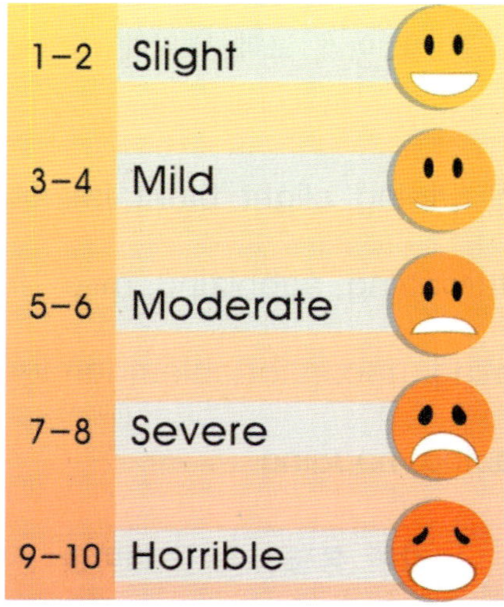

매우 강한 통증	강한 통증	경미한 통증
Agonizing, Intense, Severe, Excruciating, Raging: 지독히 아픈 **Splitting:** 쪼개질 듯이 아픈 **Searing:** 타는 듯이 아픈 **Incapacitating:** 너무 아파 일상생활이 힘든 **Jabbing:** 날카로운	**Griping:** (복부를) 콕콕 찌르는 듯 한 **Throbbing, Pulsating:** 욱신거리는	**Slight, Manageable, Uncomfortable, Mild, Subtle, Nagging:** 경미한 **Dull, Blunt:** 묵직한, 둔한 **Receding, Subsiding:** 약해지고 있는

QUIZ: 내 단어장 점검하기 !!

각각의 단어를 아래 표에 알맞게 넣으세요.

severe, pulsating, griping, slight, blunt, jabbing, subsiding, splitting, subtle, throbbing, agonizing, mild, dull, intense, searing, excruciating, uncomfortable, manageable, receding, incapacitating, raging, nagging

매우 강한 통증	강한 통증	경미한 통증

Key Expressions

통증이 얼마나 심한가요?

Q1. How bad is your pain?/Could you please tell me how bad the pain is?

A1. It's really bad. I have stabbing pain in my knee joint.

Q2. Does the headache awaken you from sleep?

A2. Yes. I couldn't sleep through the night because of my severe headache.

Q3. Is your pain severe enough to keep you awake at night?

A3. Yes, it is. I toss and turn all night due to an excruciating pain in the lower back.

Words

sleep through the night: 잠을 잘 자다

toss and turn: 엎치락뒤치락 하다

Drill: Q1-Q7을 영작하세요.

정답은 전 페이지의 Key Expressions을 참고하세요.

Q1. 통증이 얼마나 심한가요?

___

Q2. 통증이 너무 심해서 밤에 잠을 잘 수가 없나요?

___

Q3. 통증이 얼마나 심한지 말씀해 주시겠습니까?

___

Q4. 두통으로 인해 잠에서 깬 적이 있습니까?

___

Q5. 아주 심합니다. 무릎관절이 칼로 찌르는 듯이 아파요.

___

Q6. 심한 두통으로 인하여 밤에 잘 수가 없습니다.

___

Q7. 허리가 너무 아파서 밤새 엎치락뒤치락 해요.

___

Describing My Pain

Chest Pain

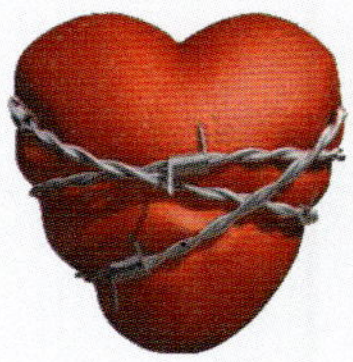

Doctor: What made you come in today?

Patient: Well, I got a pain in my chest, in my arm and also tingling in my fingers.

Doctor: I see. When did you first notice this pain?

Patient: Well, I suppose around a month ago.

Doctor: Can you describe the pain using words such as mild, moderate, severe, or the worst possible?

Patient: It's a severe pain.

Doctor: Okay. Do you think you can remember when it first came on?

Patient: Yes, I do. I had a really bad pain when I went jogging; it was so severe that I couldn't even breathe.

Doctor: And how long did it last?

Patient: Um. It lasted about ten minutes.

Doctor: I see. Now I am going to listen to your heart.
Pleaes pull up your shirt.

Words

notice: ~ 통증을 느끼다/~을 알아차리다

suppose: 아마도 ~일 것이다

come on: ~ 통증이 시작되다

go jogging: 조깅하러 가다

breathe: 숨을 쉬다

last: ~이 지속되다

pull up: ~ (옷을) 올리다

Review: 각각의 구문을 영작하세요.
정답은 전 페이지의 Dialogue를 참고하세요.

Doctor: 어디가 아프십니까?

Patient: Well, I got a pain in my chest, in my arm and also tingling in my fingers.

Doctor: 알겠습니다. 언제 통증을 처음 느끼셨습니까?

Patient: Well, I suppose around a month ago.

Doctor: 통증을 "경미한, 보통의, 심한 또는 아주 심한" 이란 단어를 사용하여 표현해 주시겠습니까?

Patient: It's a severe pain.

Doctor: 알겠습니다. 통증이 언제 처음 시작되었는지 기억나십니까?

Patient: Yes, I do. I had a really bad pain when I went jogging; it was so severe that I couldn't even breathe.

Doctor: 통증은 얼마나 오랫동안 지속되었나요?

Patient: Um. It lasted about ten minutes.

Doctor: 알겠습니다. 심장소리를 들어보겠습니다. 셔츠를 올려주세요.

Word Review: 위의 단어들을 복습하는 공간입니다.
정답은 Key Words를 참고하세요.

뜻: In English

지독히 아픈: ____________________

쪼개질 듯이 아픈: ____________________

타는 듯이 아픈: ____________________

너무 아파 일상생활이 힘든: ____________________

날카로운: ____________________

(복부를) 콕콕 찌르는 듯한: ____________________

욱신거리는: ____________________

경미한: ____________________

묵직한, 둔한: ____________________

약해지고 있는: ____________________

7. Pain Scale from 0 to 10
통증척도표 0-10

- **History of Pain Scale, 통증척도표의 역사**
  - ■ ***Code Breaker's Corner, 로리와 함께하는 미국문화 엿보기***
    - ◆ History of Pain Scale
    - ◆ Reading Material: Terrific visual communication-"how much does it hurt", 독해구문: 눈으로 말하는 위대한 대화법-"얼마나 아프세요"
    - ◆ Words, 어휘
- **Key Words for Pain Scale, 통증척도표 관련 주요어휘**
  - ■ Quiz: 내 단어장 점검하기
- **Let's make Pain Scale 0-10, 통증척도표 0-10 만들기**
- **Key Expressions, 주요구문: 통증척도표 0-10을 사용한다면 몇 점 정도 인가요?**
  - ■ Words, 어휘
  - ■ Drill, 연습문제
- **Describing My Pain: Toothache, 나의 통증 설명하기:**

치통

- Dialogue, 대화
- Words, 어휘
- Review, 복습

· **Word Review, 어휘복습**

Code Breaker's Corner: 로리와 함께 하는 미국문화 엿보기

History of Pain Scale

미국 병원에서 환자들의 통증을 가늠하기 위해 사용되는
통증척도표의 유래에 관한 간략한 글을 소개합니다.

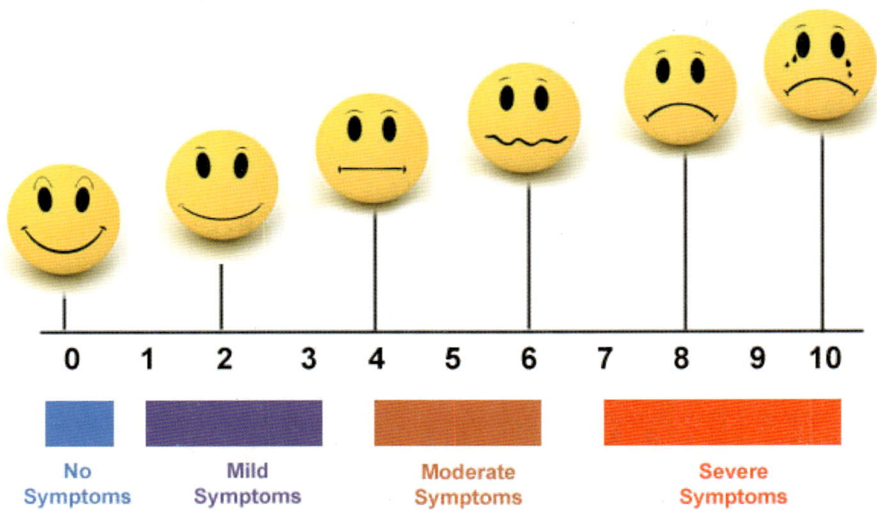

Reading Material

Terrific visual communication– "How much does it hurt?"

This description of how the pain scale was developed in the early 80s by Donna Wong, a nurse, and a child life specialist named Connie Morain Baker says that the goal was to help young children—often burn victims—who had difficulty explaining how they felt.

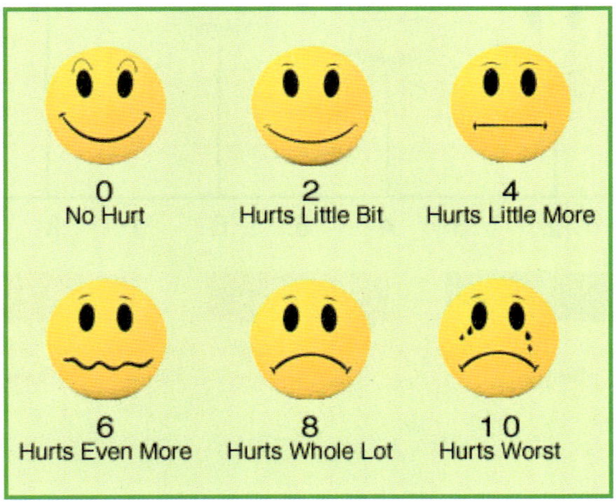
0
No Hurt
2
Hurts Little Bit
4
Hurts Little More
6
Hurts Even More
8
Hurts Whole Lot
10
Hurts Worst

Wong-Bakers Faces Pain Rating (FPR)

Wong and Baker worked with over 50 children, asking them to draw faces representing the range from "no pain" to "the worst pain they could imagine."

They used the then-popular "smiley face" stickers as a starting point. They got drawings like these, showing a wide range of detail in the faces.

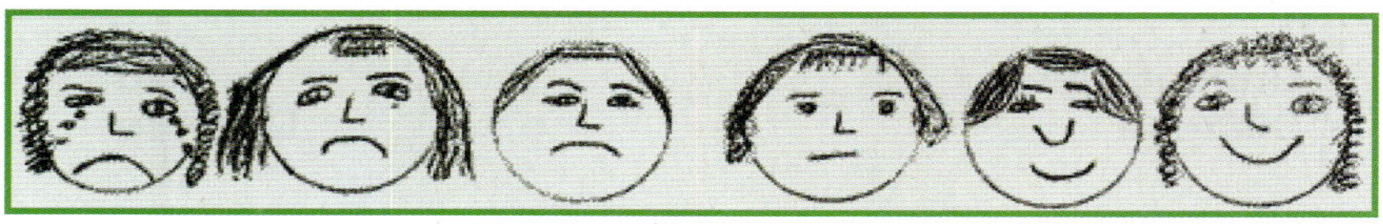

A professional artist later created the simpler faces for the scale. The artist created more variations among the eyebrows on the faces but otherwise used what the kids created.

Source: www.awdsgn.com/dailyjourn

Words

specialist: 전문의

burn victims: 화상을 입은 환자들

difficulty explaining: 설명하는 것에 어려움을 겪다.

then-popular: 그 당시 인기 있던

eyebrows: 눈썹

That was then, this is now: 그때는 그때이고 지금은 지금이다.

Key Words for Pain Scale

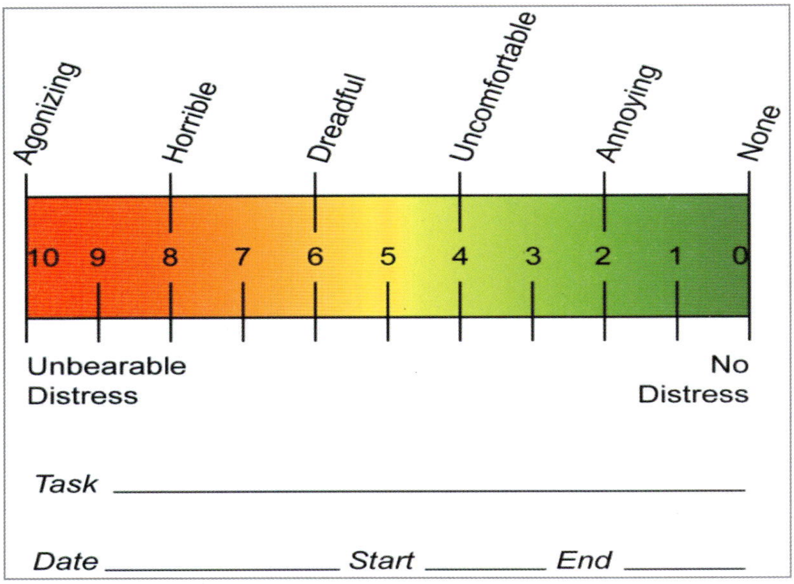

0-None, No distress: 무통

2-Annoying, Tender: 통증으로 인해 짜증이 나는 정도

4-Uncomfortable, Nagging, Aching: 몸과 마음이 불편할 정도의 통증

6-Dreadful, Gnawing: 지독한

8-Horrible: 끔찍한 통증

9-Unbearable distress: 참을 수 없는 고통

10-Agonizing: 극도의 고통

Distress: 고통, 괴로움

QUIZ: 내 단어장 점검하기 !!

아래 단어 및 문장을 읽고 알맞은 통증의 이름을 적어보세요.

No distress: ....

Annoying: ....

Uncomfortable: ....

Dreadful: ....

Horrible: ....

Unbearable distress: ....

Agonizing: ....

Distress: ....

Let's Make Pain Scale 0-10

아래의 통증관련 어휘들을 **Pain Scale 0-10**에 통증의 정도에 따라 배열 하세요.

Horrible, Unbearable distress, Excruciating, Manageable, Throbbing, Dull, Aching, Nagging, Tender, Blunt, Gnawing, Gripping, Agonizing,

Pain Scale 0-10

0	1-2	3	4	5
No Pain				

6	7	8	9	10 The worst possible

Key Expressions

통증척도표 0-10을 사용한다면,
통증이 몇 점 정도인가요?

Q1. Using a scale of 1 to 10, how would you rate your pain right now?

A1. I would have to say mine is an 8, and I am always in pain. I don't know what it is like to be without this pain, anymore. I have been like this for the last 10 years.

Q2. What is your pain level today?/what is your pain quotient today?

A2. I can say it is about 11. I am dying here.

Q3. On a pain scale of 1-10 with one being the lowest level and ten being the highest level, how much pain are you experiencing right now?

A3. Even though I have a very high pain threshold, I would say around nine and a half (9 1/2).

Words

high pain threshold: 통증을 느끼는 최고치

pain quotient: 통증수치

Drill: Q1-Q6을 영작하세요.

정답은 전 페이지의 Key Expressions을 참고하세요.

Q1. 통증척도표 1-10을 사용한다면, 지금 몇 점 정도의 통증을 느끼나요?

____

Q2. 1점이 가장 적은 통증이고 10점이 가장 큰 통증인 통증척도표 1-10에서 환자분의 통증수치는 몇 점 정도입니까?

____

Q3. 오늘은 통증을 얼마나 느끼십니까?

____

Q4. 약 11점입니다. 아파서 죽을 것만 같아요.

____

Q5. 나의 통증은 8점 정도이며 항상 통증이 있습니다.

____

Q6. 나는 통증을 느끼는 최고치가 상당히 높은 편이지만, 통증이 9.5 점 정도가 되는 것 같습니다.

____

Describing My Pain

Toothache

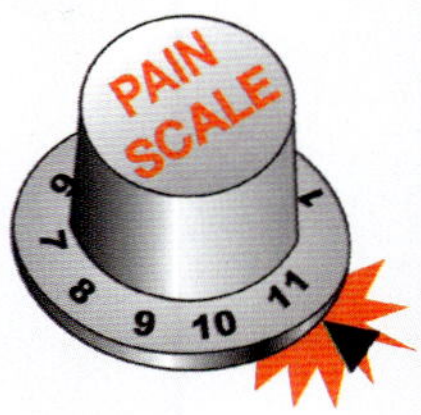

Doctor: How long does each episode of toothache usually last?

Patient: It usually lasts for half an hour.

Doctor: When was the first time you noticed it?

Patient: Well, I noticed that one of my molar teeth was hurting me four days ago.

Doctor: Could you describe your pain, please?

Patient: It's a severe stabbing pain.

Doctor: If you describe your pain from 1 to 10, where would you be on the pain scale?

Patient: I think about 1000 if it was available.

Doctor: Oh! What makes the pain worse?

Patient: I guess after eating sweet things, it gets worse.

Doctor: First, we need to take an X-ray of your teeth to check whether you have a cavity.

Words

each episode of toothache: 치통을 느낄 때마다

molar tooth: 어금니

TIP

충치:

a cavity
tooth decay
dental caries

I have a sweet tooth.: 나는 단 것을 좋아해요.

Review: 각각의 구문을 영작하세요.
정답은 전 페이지의 Dialogue를 참고하세요.

Doctor: 치통이 시작되면 얼마나 오랫동안 지속되나요?

____

Patient: It usually lasts for half an hour.

Doctor: 언제 처음 알게 되었지요?

____

Patient: Well, I noticed that one of my molar teeth was hurting me four days ago.

Doctor: 어떤 통증인지 설명해 주시겠어요?

____

Patient: It's a severe stabbing pain.

Doctor: 만일 통증을 1-10으로 표현한다면, 몇 점 정도일까요?

____

Patient: I think about 1000 if it was available.

Doctor: 오! 무엇이 통증을 악화시키나요?

____

Patient: I guess after eating sweet things, it gets worse.

Doctor: 우선, 충치가 있는지 확인하기 위해 엑스레이를 찍겠습니다.

____

Word Review: 위의 단어들을 복습하는 공간입니다.
정답은 Key Words를 참고하세요.

뜻: In English

무통: ______________________

통증으로 인해 짜증이 나는 정도: ______________________

몸과 마음이 불편할 정도의 통증: ______________________

지독한 통증: ______________________

끔찍한 통증: ______________________

참을 수 없는 고통: ______________________

극도의 고통: ______________________

고통, 괴로움: ______________________

8. Duration of pain
통증의 지속시간

- **Key Words, 주요어휘**
    - Quiz: 내 단어장 점검하기
- **Key Expressions, 주요구문: 통증이 지속적인가요 또는 간헐적인가요?**
    - Words, 어휘
    - Drill, 연습문제
- **Describing My Pain: Seasonal Allergy, 나의 통증 설명하기: 계절성 앨러지**
    - Dialogue, 대화
    - Words, 어휘
    - Review, 복습
- **Word Review, 어휘복습**

Key Words

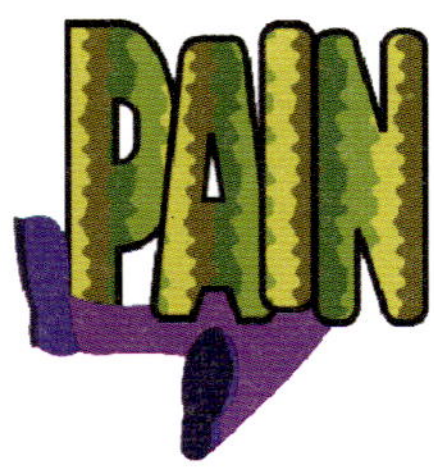

서서히 오는 통증 VS 갑작스러운 통증	지속적인 통증 VS 일시적인, 간헐적인 통증
Gradual pain: 서서히 오는 통증 --- **Sudden pain:** 갑작스러운 통증	**Constant pain,** **Persistent pain,** **Continuous pain,** **Gnawing pain:** 지속적인 통증 --- **Transient pain,** **Intermittent pain,** **Come and go,** **On and off,** **Sporadic:** 일시적인, 간헐적인 통증

QUIZ: 내 단어장 점검하기 !!

아래 단어 및 문장을 읽고 알맞은 통증의 이름을 적어보세요.

Constant pain: ....

Intermittent pain: ....

Gradual pain: ....

Sporadic: ....

Sudden pain: ....

Gnawing pain: ....

Transient pain: ....

Come and go: ....

On and off: ....

Continuous pain: ....

Persistent pain: ....

Key Expressions

통증이 지속적인가요 또는 간헐적인가요?

Q1. When your pain started, did it come on suddenly, or did it start out gradually?/When the pain occurred, did it happen suddenly or develop gradually?

A1. Mine came on suddenly, out of the blue.

Q2. Is your neck pain constant or does it come and go?/Is it persistent or on and off?

A2. It comes and goes./Well, it's persistent. I have had this pain for more than three years.

Q3. When the pain began, did it start suddenly?

A3. Yes. It flared up suddenly.

Words

out of the blue: 예기치 못한

flares up: 통증이 급작스럽게 더 심해지다.

Drill: Q1-Q7을 영작하세요.

정답은 전 페이지의 Key Expressions을 참고하세요.

Q1. 통증이 시작될 때 갑작스럽게 아팠나요 아니면 서서히 아팠나요?

Q2. 목의 통증이 지속적인가요 아니면 간헐적인가요?

Q3. 통증이 갑자기 시작됐나요?

Q4. 간헐적입니다.

Q5. 예기치 못하게 갑작스럽게 아프기 시작했어요.

Q6. 갑자기 아주 심하게 통증이 시작됐습니다.

Q7. 항상 통증을 느낍니다. 3년 이상 이 통증이 계속되고 있습니다.

Describing My Pain

Seasonal Allergy

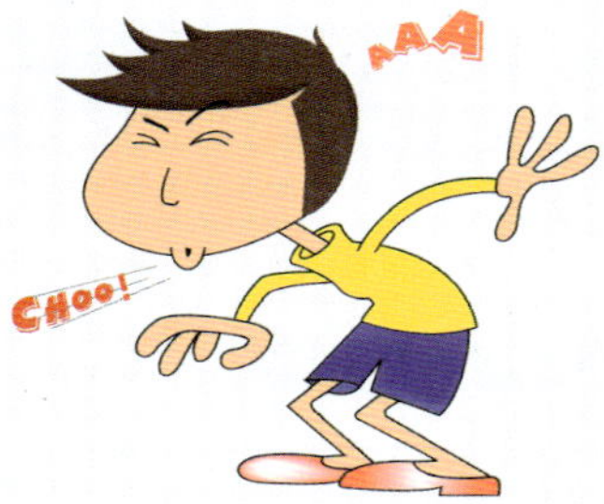

Doctor: Have you had any other symptoms with your seasonal allergy?
Patient: Yes. I had a migraine.

Doctor: Could you describe your migraine please?
Patient: Well, it's like a stabbing pain.

Doctor: Which side of your head is most affected?
Patient: The left side of my temple is hurting me badly.

Doctor: Can you think of any other symptoms that happened when migraine started?
Patient: Well, I have had blurred vision in both of my eyes which lasts for about an hour or so.

Doctor: Does your migraine come and go or do you have it all the time?
Patient: It comes and goes.

Doctor: Is it worse at a certain time of the day?
Patient: Yes. I think it becomes a lot worse in the morning.

Words

seasonal allergy: 계절성 앨러지

migraine/migraine headache: 편두통

temple: 관자놀이

affected area: 아픈 부위

blurred vision: 흐릿한 시야

TIP

만성통증 vs 급성통증

Chronic pain (used for describing pain that is serious and lasts for a long time**):**

만성통증은 오랫동안 지속되는 심각한 통증을 의미함

Acute pain (used for describing pain that is very strong and sharp and lasts only for a short time**):** 급성통증은 짧은 순간 동안 지속되는 매우 강하며 예리한 통증을 의미함

Review: 각각의 구문을 영작하세요.
정답은 전 페이지의 Dialogue를 참고하세요.

Doctor: 계절성 앨러지와 수반되는 다른 증상이 있습니까?

____

Patient: Yes. I had a migraine.

Doctor: 당신의 편두통이 어떤지 설명해 주시겠습니까?

____

Patient: Well, it's like a stabbing pain.

Doctor: 머리의 어느 부위가 가장 아프십니까?

____

Patient: The left side of my temple is hurting me badly.

Doctor: 편두통이 시작될 때 수반되었던 다른 증상을 말씀해 주시겠습니까?

____

Patient: Well, I have had blurred vision in both of my eyes which lasts for about an hour or so.

Doctor: 편두통이 간헐적인가요 또는 지속적인가요?

____

Patient: It comes and goes.

Doctor: 편두통이 특정한 시간대에 악화되나요?

____

Patient: Yes. I think it becomes a lot worse in the morning.

Word Review: 위의 단어들을 복습하는 공간입니다.
정답은 Key Words를 참고하세요.

뜻: In English

서서히 오는 통증: ____________________

갑작스러운 통증: ____________________

지속적인 통증: ____________________

____

일시적인, 간헐적인 통증: ____________________

____

9. Precipitating Factors
통증을 야기시키는 원인

- **Key Words, 주요어휘**
    - ■ Quiz: 내 단어장 점검하기
- **Key Expressions, 주요구문:**

통증이 처음 시작될 때 무엇을 하고 계셨나요?

- ◆ Words, 어휘
- ◆ Drill, 연습문제

통증을 야기시키는 특별한 것이 있나요?

- ◆ Words, 어휘
- ◆ Drill, 연습문제

- **Describing My Pain: Upset Stomach, 나의 통증 설명하기: 속 쓰림**
    - ■ Dialogue, 대화
    - ■ Words, 어휘
    - ■ Review, 복습
- **Word Review, 어휘복습**

Key Words

Food Related Precipitating Factors: 통증을 유발하는 음식과 관련된 요소	Other Precipitating Factors: 통증을 유발하는 기타 다른 요소
Spicy food: 향신료가 첨가된 음식 **Skipping meals:** 식사를 거름 **Eating certain foods such as cheese, alcohol, chocolate, coffee, peanuts, MSG or red wine:** 치즈, 술, 초콜릿, 커피, 땅콩, 화학조미료 또는 와인과 같은 특정 음식의 섭취	**Certain movements:** 특정한 동작 **Bright lights:** 밝은 빛 **Loud noises:** 시끄러운 소리 **Strong odors:** 강한 냄새 **Physical or emotional stress:** 신체적 또는 정신적 스트레스 **Changes in sleep patterns:** 수면시간이 바뀜 **Exposure to smoke:** 담배연기에 노출 **Selected medications:** 다른 특정 약품

QUIZ: 내 단어장 점검하기 !!

아래 단어 및 문장을 읽고 알맞은 통증의 이름을 적어보세요.

Physical or emotional stress: ....

Bright lights: ....

Strong odors: ....

Skipping meals: ....

Spicy food: ....

Changes in sleep patterns: ....

Loud noises: ....

Exposure to smoke: ....

Selected medications: ....

Certain movements: ....

Eating certain foods such as cheese, alcohol, chocolate, coffee, peanuts, MSG or red wine: ....

....

....

Key Expressions

통증이 처음 시작될 때 무엇을 하고 계셨나요?

Q1. What were you doing when your pain began?

A1. I was going up the stairs.

Q2. What were you doing when your lower backache started?

A2. I was taking the garbage out.

Q3. What were you doing just before the pain began?

A3. I was lifting heavy objects.

Words

going up the stairs: 계단을 오르다

taking the garbage out: 쓰레기를 버리다

lifting heavy objects: 무거운 것을 들다

Drill: Q1-Q6을 영작하세요.

정답은 전 페이지의 Key Expressions을 참고하세요.

Q1. 통증이 시작될 때 무엇을 하고 계셨나요?

____

Q2. 요통이 시작될 때 무엇을 하고 계셨나요?

____

Q3. 통증이 시작되기 전에 무엇을 하고 계셨나요?

____

Q4. 계단을 오르고 있었어요.

____

Q5. 쓰레기를 버리고 있었습니다.

____

Q6. 무거운 것을 들고 있었습니다.

____

Key Expressions

통증을 야기시키는 특별한 것이 있나요?

Q1. What triggers your pain?/What do you think cause the pain?/Does anything specific trigger your pain?

A1. I can't say that one thing causes my pain.

Q2. Are there any foods that precipitate the pain?/Are there any foods that you think may bring on the pain?

A2. I think whenever I drink red wine, it seems to come on.

Q3. Are there any precipitating factors for your cluster headaches?

A3. Well, I think they seem to come on whenever I drink caffeinated beverages.

Words

trigger: ~을 야기 시키다

come on: (통증이) 시작되다

cluster headaches: 군집성 두통

Drill: Q1-Q6을 영작하세요.

정답은 전 페이지의 Key Expressions를 참고하세요.

Q1. 무엇이 통증을 야기시키나요?

Q2. 통증을 야기시키는 음식이 있나요?

Q3. 군집성 두통을 야기시키는 음식이 있나요?

Q4. 내 생각에는 적포도주를 마실 때마다 편두통이 오는 것 같아요.

Q5. 내가 카페인이 든 음료를 섭취할 때마다 두통이 발생되는 것 같아요.

Q6. 무엇이 통증을 야기시키는지 모르겠습니다.

Describing My Pain

Upset Stomach

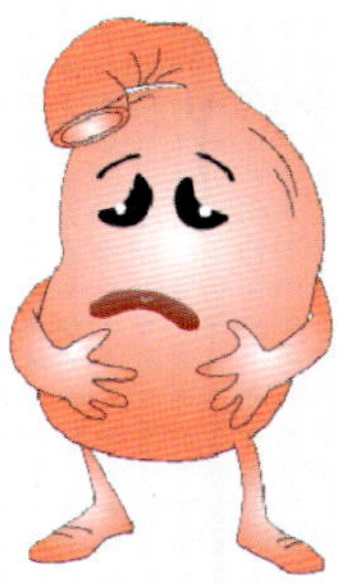

Doctor: Good Morning, Mr. Smith. I am an attending physician here at the international medical center. How can I help you today?

Mr. Smith: I have a very bad stomachache.

Doctor: Can you tell me about your pain, please?

Mr. Smith: Well, it's like a stabbing pain here in my upper abdomen.

Doctor: Have you eaten anything that might have upset your stomach?

Mr. Smith: Actually, I had some beer last night, but not much.

Doctor: Does anything else make the pain worse?

Mr. Smith: I think whenever I eat hot and spicy food, my stomach hurts a lot.

Doctor: I see. I am going to examine your belly. For that I need you to lie down on the examination table. Let me help you.
Mr. Smith: Thanks.

Doctor: No problem. Are you comfortable?
Mr. Smith: Yes, I am.

Doctor: I will listen to your bowel sounds first. Would you please raise your gown up?
Mr. Smith: Like this?

Doctor: Yes. Mr. Smith, now I am going to press your belly first lightly and then deeply, please let me know if it hurts or makes you feel uncomfortable.
Mr. Smith: Ouch! Right side of my belly. It hurts badly.

Doctor: I'm sorry. Now, I'll press in & release. Please let me know if it hurts when I press in or when I let go.
Mr. Smith: Alright.

Doctor: One last thing. I'll tap on different parts of your belly, so please let me know if it hurts.
Mr. Smith: Okay.

Words

upset stomach: 속 쓰림

stabbing pain: 칼로 찌르는 듯한 통증

upper abdomen: 복부 위쪽, 상 복부

upset your stomach: 위를 자극하다

hot and spicy: 맵고 자극적인(뜨겁다는 온도의 개념은 포함되지 않음).

TIP

재발하다

Recur
Acting up again
Flare up again

Review: 각각의 구문을 영작하세요.
정답은 전 페이지의 Dialogue를 참고하세요.

Doctor: Good Morning, Mr. Smith. I am an attending physician here at the international medical center. How can I help you today?
Mr. Smith: I have a very bad stomachache.

Doctor: 어떻게 아프신지 설명해 주시겠습니까?

Mr. Smith: Well, it's like a stabbing pain here in my upper abdomen.

Doctor: 위를 자극할 만한 음식을 드셨나요?

Mr. Smith: Actually, I had some beer last night, but not much.

Doctor: 통증을 악화시키는 것이 있습니까?

Mr. Smith: I think whenever I eat hot and spicy food, my stomach hurts a lot.

Doctor: 알겠습니다. 복부를 검사하겠습니다. 그러기 위해서는 여기 검사대에 누우셔야 합니다.

Let me help you.
Mr. Smith: Thanks.

Doctor: No problem. Are you comfortable?

Mr. Smith: Yes, I am.

Doctor: 복부청진을 하겠습니다. 가운을 올려주시겠습니까?

____

Mr. Smith: Like this?

Doctor: 예. 스미스 선생님, 이제 복부를 살짝 누른 후 세게 누르겠습니다. 눌렀을 때 아프거나 불편함을 느끼시면 말씀해 주세요.

____

____

Mr. Smith: Ouch! Right side of my belly. It hurts badly.

Doctor: I'm sorry.

이제 꾸욱 눌렀다가 떼겠습니다. 꾸욱 눌렀을 때 아픈지 아니면 떼었을 때 아픈지 말씀해 주세요.

____

Mr. Smith: Alright.

Doctor: 마지막으로 복부의 여러 부위를 두드리겠습니다. 만일 아프시면 말씀하세요.

____

____

Mr. Smith: Okay

Word Review: 위의 단어들을 복습하는 공간입니다.
정답은 Key Words를 참고하세요.

뜻: In English

밝은 빛: ____________________

시끄러운 소리: ____________________

강한 냄새: ____________________

신체적 또는 정신적 스트레스: ____________________

수면시간이 바뀜: ____________________

담배연기에 노출: ____________________

식사를 거름: ____________________

치즈, 술, 초콜릿, 커피, 땅콩, 화학조미료 또는 와인과 같은 특정 음식의 섭취: ____________________

____

다른 특정 약품: ____________________

특정한 동작: ____________________

향신료가 첨가된 음식: ____________________

10. Alleviation & Aggravation of Pain
통증의 완화 및 악화

- **Key Words, 주요어휘**
  - ■ Quiz: 내 단어장 점검하기

- **Key Expressions, 주요구문:**

무엇이 통증을 완화 시키나요?

◆ Words, 어휘

◆ Drill, 연습문제

무엇이 통증을 악화시키나요?

◆ Words, 어휘

◆ Drill, 연습문제

통증이 점점 완화 또는 악화 되나요?

◆ Words, 어휘

◆ Drill, 연습문제

- **Describing My Pain: Cluster Headaches, 나의 통증 설명하기: 군집성 두통**
  - ■ Dialogue, 대화
  - ■ Words, 어휘
  - ■ Review, 복습

- **Word Review, 어휘복습**

Key Words

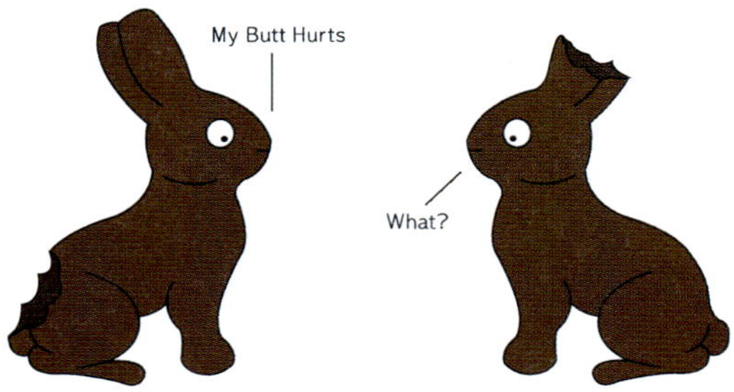

Feel better, Relieve: 완화되다	Aggravate, Get worse: 악화되다
Alleviating factors: **완화시키는 요소** By lying down: 눕기 Rest: 휴식 Standing: 서있기 Stretch: 스트레칭 Pain medication: 진통제 복용 Putting something hot/cold on it: 따뜻한 것/차가운 것 대고 있기 Exercise: 운동	**Aggravating factors:** **악화시키는 요소** Eating certain foods: 특정한 음식을 섭취 A repetitive motion: 반복되는 동작 Lifting, Pulling or Pushing heavy objects: 무거운 것 들기, 밀거나 당기기 Too much exercise: 심한 운동 Not enough exercise: 운동부족 Staying in one position for too long: 너무 오랫동안 한 자세를 취함 The weather: 날씨의 영향

QUIZ: 내 단어장 점검하기 !!

각각의 단어를 아래 표에 알맞게 넣으세요.

Feel better, Relieve: 완화되다	Aggravate, Get worse: 악화되다
Alleviating factors:	**Aggravating factors:**
By lying down:	Eating certain foods:
Rest:	A repetitive motion:
Standing:	Lifting, Pulling or Pushing heavy objects:
Stretch:	Too much exercise:
Pain medication:	Not enough exercise:
Putting something hot/cold on it:	Staying in one position for too long:
Exercise:	The weather:

Key Expressions

무엇이 통증을 완화 시키나요?

Q1. If you take a pain medication, does it help to relieve your arthritis pain?

A1. Yes, it does. If I take an analgesic, my arthritis pain stops for a while.

Q2. Does anything make you feel better?/Is there anything that makes you feel better when you are in pain?/Is there anything you do that makes the pain easy?

A2. Yes. If I sit or lay down for a while then I feel much better. Also, changing my position from sitting to standing up helps relieve my pain, too.

Q3. If you use a heating pad or ice pack, does that help lessen your pain?

A3. Of course. Heating pad works for me greatly.

Words

analgesic: 진통제

arthritis: 관절염

heating pad: 온 찜질

Drill: Q1-Q7을 영작하세요.

정답은 전 페이지의 Key Expressions를 참고하세요

Q1. 진통제를 복용하면 관절통증이 완화되나요?

____

Q2. 통증을 완화시키는 것이 있습니까?

____

Q3. 온 찜질이나 냉 찜질을 하면, 통증완화에 도움이 되나요?

____

Q4 진통제를 복용하면, 관절통증이 멈춥니다

____

Q5. 온 찜질이 특히 좋아요.

____

Q6. 만일 내가 한참 동안 앉거나 누워있으면, 훨씬 더 나아져요.

____

Q7. 앉은 자세에서 서있는 자세로 바꾸면 통증이 완화 되요.

____

Key Expressions

무엇이 통증을 악화시키나요?

Q1. Does anything make the pain worse?/Does anything specific make your pain worse?

A1. Yes. If I sit or stay in one position for too long then, I feel a lot of pain in my back and hip.

Q2. Does coffee make your headache worse?

A2. Not really.

Q3. What makes your pain worse?

A3. The rain and cold can aggravate my pain. To make matters worse, my pain meds are barely working on those days.

Words

to make matters worse: 설상가상으로

pain meds: 진통제

barely: 거의 ~하지 않다.

aggravate: ~을 악화시키다

Drill: Q1-Q6을 영작하세요.

정답은 전 페이지의 Key Expressions를 참고하세요

Q1. 통증을 악화시키는 것이 있습니까?

____

Q2. 커피가 두통을 악화시키나요?

____

Q3. 무엇이 통증을 악화시키나요?

____

Q4. 만일 같은 자세로 오래 앉아있거나 서 있으면 허리와 엉덩이 부위에 심한 통증을 느낍니다.

____

Q5. 설상가상으로 그런 날에는 진통제도 거의 듣지 않습니다.

____

Q6. 비가 오거나 날씨가 추워지면 통증이 더 심해집니다.

____

Key Expressions

통증이 점점 완화 또는 악화 되나요?

Q1. Has your pain been getting worse over time or has it stayed about the same?

A1. Actually, it has been getting progressively worse over the past two weeks.

Q2. Are the headaches increasing in severity?

A2. Yes, they are.

Q3. Is your pain worse at a certain time of the day?

A3. Yes. The pain is usually persistent, but it gets worse at night.

Words

progressively: 점차적으로

severity: 세기, 강도

persistent: 지속적인

Drill: Q1-Q5를 영작하세요.

정답은 전 페이지의 Key Expressions를 참고하세요

Q1. 통증이 시간이 지나면서 계속 더 악화가 됐나요, 아니면 거의 같은 정도인가요?

___

Q2. 두통이 점점 더 심해지나요?

___

Q3. 통증이 하루 중 특별한 시간대에 더 악화되나요?

___

Q4. 사실, 지난 두 주간 점차적으로 악화되고 있습니다.

___

Q5. 계속 통증을 느끼지만, 밤이 되면 더 심하게 아파져요.

___

Describing My Pain

Cluster headaches

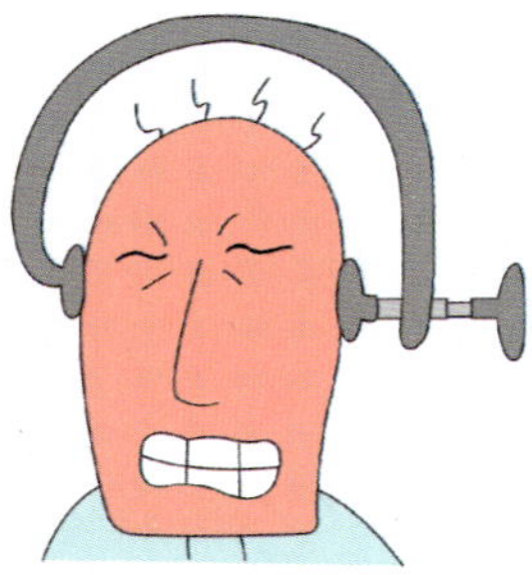

Dr. Park: Well, on the chart, you have very bad headaches. Can you describe the pain? How does your headache feel?

Mr. Jung: It's stabbing and excruciating.

Dr. Park: Alright. On a pain scale of 1-10 with 1 being the least and 10 being the worst pain, how would you rate it right now?

Mr. Jung: I would say about 9. Over the past 3-4 days I had experienced the worst pain in my life. It was horrible.

Dr. Park: And how long does your headache usually last?

Mr. Jung: Well, it seems to vary. It usually lasts a day and it wears off in the second half of the day. But last week, it completely immobilized me.

Dr. Park: I see. And where is the pain generally located?

Mr. Jung: Well, the pain is usually on the right side of my head, but it never occurs on both sides.

Dr. Park: Does it radiate anywhere?
Mr. Jung: No, I don't think so, although it's often around my eye and cheek on the same side.

Dr. Park: You said, only right side of your head is affected, and it is around your eye and cheek on the same side, right?
Mr. Jung: That's correct, Doctor.

Dr. Park: Can you show me exactly where it hurts with your finger?
Mr. Jung: Right here, doctor… and right over here, too.

Dr. Park: I got it. So, the pain is mainly at the front of your head and it involves a forehead, right side of your temple, eye and cheek.
Mr. Jung: That's right. Fortunately, I don't have any pain in the back of my head.

Dr. Park: Are there any foods that precipitate the pain? What I mean is if there are any foods that may bring on or trigger the headaches.
Mr. Jung: Um, I think whenever I drink caffeinated beverages like coffee, the pain seems to come on.

Dr. Park: So, you mentioned coffee! Then, is there anything that makes you feel better when you are in pain?

Mr. Jung: Not that I know of. Even the strong pain meds don't work for my headaches. Do you have any idea of what's going on with me?

Dr. Park: Well, Mr. Jung. I have some thoughts. You are suffering from cluster headaches. The cluster headaches occur predominantly in young male around 30's and affects only one side of the head, right or left. Mr. Jung, first of all, you should avoid caffeinated beverages from now on because it is one of the precipitating factors for your headache.

Mr. Jung: Then, I will not drink any coffee and caffeinated beverages at all.

Words

immobilize: 거동을 못하게 하다

the second half of the day: 오후

selected foods: 특정음식

temple: 관자놀이

predominantly: 주로

caffeinated beverage: 카페인이 들어있는 음료

Review: 각각의 구문을 영작하세요.
정답은 전 페이지의 Dialogue를 참고하세요.

Dr. Park: Well, on the chart, you have very bad headaches.

그럼 통증을 설명해 주시겠습니까? 어떤 두통입니까?

Mr. Jung: 예리한 것으로 찌르는 듯하며 참을 수 없을 정도로 심합니다.

Dr. Park: 알겠습니다. 1점은 가장 통증이 약하고 10점이 통증이 가장 심한 1~10의 통증척도표를 사용한다면, 현재 통증이 몇 점 정도가 될까요?

Mr. Jung: 9점 정도요.

지난 3-4일 동안 내가 겪은 통증은 평생 겪어본 통증에서 가장 심한 통증이었습니다.

아주 끔찍했습니다.

Dr. Park: 통증이 얼마나 지속되나요?

Mr. Jung: 음. 일정하지는 않아요.

주로 하루 동안 아프지만 오후에는 통증이 잦아듭니다.

But last week, it completely immobilized me.

Dr. Park: 알겠습니다. 주로 어느 부위가 아픈가요?

Mr. Jung: 머리 오른쪽 부분이 주로 아파요. 하지만 결코 머리 양쪽 부분이 모두 아프지는 않아요.

Dr. Park: 통증이 다른 곳으로도 옮겨가나요?

Mr. Jung: No, I don't think so, although it's often around my eye and cheek on the same side.

Dr. Park: 머리 오른쪽 부위만 아프고 같은 쪽의 눈 주위와 뺨이 아프다고 했지요, 그렇지요?

Mr. Jung: That's correct, Doctor.

Dr. Park: 아픈 부위를 손가락으로 가리켜 주시겠습니까?

Mr. Jung: Right here, doctor… and right over here, too.

Dr. Park: I got it. So, the pain is mainly at the front of your head and it involves a forehead, right side of your temple, eye and cheek.

Mr. Jung: That's right.

다행히도 머리 뒷 부분은 아프지 않습니다.

Dr. Park: 통증을 야기시키는 음식이 있습니까?

제 말은 두통을 일으키는 특정 음식이 있느냐는 것입니다.

Mr. Jung: 음. 제 생각에는 커피와 같이 카페인이 들어 있는 음료를 마실 때 두통이 생기는 것 같습니다.

Dr. Park: So, you mentioned coffee!

그러면 아플 때 통증을 완화시켜주는 것이 있습니까?

Mr. Jung: Not that I know of. Even the strong pain meds don't work for my headaches. Do you have any idea of what's going on with me?

Dr. Park: Well, Mr. Jung. I have some thoughts.

군집성 두통을 앓고 있습니다.

The cluster headaches occur predominantly in young male around 30's and affects only one side of the head, right or left.

환자분(MR. Jung)은 우선 카페인이든 음료를 금해야 합니다.

왜냐하면 환자분의 두통을 야기시키는 요소들 중 하나가 카페인이 든

음료이기 때문입니다.

Mr. Jung: Then, I will not drink any coffee and caffeinated beverages at all.

Word Review: 위의 단어들을 복습하는 공간입니다.
정답은 Key Words를 참고하세요.

뜻: In English

완화되다:______________________________

악화되다:______________________________

심한 운동: ______________________________

무거운 것 들기, 밀거나 당기기:______________________________

휴식/서있기/눕기:______________________________

운동부족:______________________________

스트레칭/운동:______________________________

반복되는 동작:______________________________

날씨의 영향:______________________________

특정한 음식을 섭취:______________________________

너무 오랫동안 한 자세를 취함:______________________________

진통제 복용:______________________________

악화시키는 요소:______________________________

완화시키는 요소:______________________________

따뜻한 것 대고 있기: ______________________________

차가운 것 대고 있기:______________________________

11. How to Write A Pain Journal
통증일지 작성법

· **Drill, 연습문제**

Drill

아래의 통증일지의 빈칸을 영작해 보세요.

How to Write a Pain Journal (통증일지 작성법)							
Date	**When did your pain begin?**	**Where did you feel the pain?**	**What were you doing?**	**What does it feel like?**	**How bad is your pain on a scale 0-10?**	**How long did it last?**	**What did you try to make it better?**
06/16	Late morning	In my lower back	Working out	Sharp	8	Half an hour	Took my medication & took a rest
06/17	Around midnight	Left side of my temple	Trying to fall asleep	Throbbin g	3	A couple of hours	Took a pain medication

12. 정답 및 해석

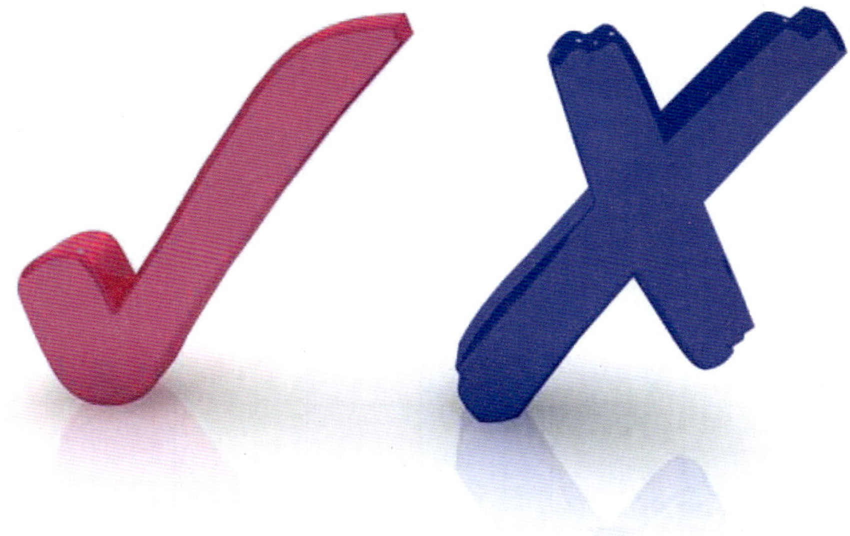

1. 통증의 성질(종류)
주요어휘

C. 쪼는 듯한 통증

위에서 느끼는 작열감 또는 쪼는 듯한 통증으로 주로 위궤양과 동반되며 30분-3시간 가량 지속됩니다.

D. 타는 듯한 통증

마치 신체의 일부가 뜨거운 것을 만진 것과 같은 느낌입니다.

E. 근육통이 있는, 몸이 쑤시는

팔이 쑤셔요.

마라톤을 뛰고 난 후 다리근육이 너무 쑤셔요.

F. 피부가 벗겨져(까져서) 쓰라린

신발에 쓸린 그녀의 발은 군데군데 피부가 벗겨져 있었습니다.

나는 잇몸과 연구개 부위가 쓰라립니다.

G. 만졌을 때 또는 촉진 시 느끼는 통증

눌렀을 때 느끼는 통증은 증상이 있는 부위를 만졌을 때 느끼는 통증입니다.

I. 콕콕 찌르는 듯한 통증

날카로운 물질이 피부에 구멍을 뚫음으로써 생기는 따끔한 통증입니다.

J. 묵직하게 지속적으로 아픈 통증

심하지는 않지만 오래도록 지속되는 통증입니다.

지속적이며 불쾌하지만 주로 강하지 않은 통증입니다.

K. 방사통

방사통은 통증의 진원지에서 신체의 다른 부분으로 퍼져나가는 통증입니다.

L. 저릿저릿한 감각

발이 저려요.

1. 통증의 종류
주요어휘 연습문제 정답

J	O	M	R	B	T	S	F	I	Q	T	U	R	S	T	V	N	S
E	F	M	A	S	B	R	D	V	Y	W	M	V	Y	D	O	T	P
X	J	T	D	O	U	P	Y	G	M	I	C	R	P	O	I	V	A
C	O	N	I	R	R	Q	J	K	U	T	Q	I	E	N	M	U	B
R	N	C	A	E	N	Q	G	V	H	J	T	I	G	T	P	H	O
U	A	W	T	N	I	T	M	T	Q	F	E	I	E	A	U	C	P
C	Q	B	I	E	N	G	L	P	A	X	N	W	A	E	H	O	M
I	L	S	O	S	G	N	R	K	O	G	D	W	Q	N	Q	S	N
A	P	I	N	S		A	N	D		N	E	E	D	L	E	S	Q
T	U	R		N	S	W	V	S	M	A	R	T		P	A	I	N
I	X	R	P	F	E	I	E	C	B	K	N	H	X	L	G	N	W
N	B	I	A	R	N	N	F	A	N	N	E	R	G	S	H	W	C
G	J	H	I	W	S	G	S	B	V	O	S	O	L	G	R	R	C
	D	H	N	A	A		I	Y	R	G	S	B	B	P	E	F	V
P	I	T	T	J	T	P	Q	X	Q	G	R	B	B	J	N	M	H
A	Y	I	G	L	I	A	C	A	D	K	P	I	H	Q	U	V	C
I	O	R	A	C	O	I	Y	R	K	L	E	N	R	W	E	W	V
N	C	Y	G	A	N	N	U	Q	W	S	N	G	J	R	P	O	Q

Excruciating pain	Smart pain	Gnawing pain
Burning sensation	Soreness	Raw
Tenderness	Stinging sensation	Radiation pain
Pins and needles	Throbbing	

2. 통증부위
주요구문 해석

어느 부위가 아프세요?

Q1. 어느 부위가 아프세요?

A1. 지난 밤부터 배의 오른쪽 위 부위가 심하게 아파요.

Q2. 통증이 한 곳에서 시작되어 다른 곳으로 퍼지나요?

A2. 예. 통증이 목에서 시작해서 왼쪽 팔로 옮겨 가요.

Q3. 표면이 아픈가요 아니면 속에서 통증을 느끼나요?

A3. 겉이 아니고 속에서 아픈 것 같아요.

Q4. 몸의 한 부위가 아픈가요, 아니면 여러 곳이 아픈가요?

A4. 이유 없이 온몸이 다 심하게 아파요.

Q5. 한쪽 부위만 아픈가요 또는 양쪽 부위 다 아픈가요?

A5. 이상한 통증이 턱의 한 쪽 부위에서만 느껴져요.

Q6. 어디가 가장 아프세요?

A6. 오른쪽 허벅지에 통증이 느껴져요.

2. 통증부위
나의 통증 설명하기

목의 통증

Doctor: 어디가 아프셔서 오셨어요?

Patient: 음, 나는 하루 평균 8-10시간을 컴퓨터 앞에서 일을 합니다. 그런데 요즘 목에 통증을 느낍니다.

Doctor: 통증을 설명해 주시겠습니까?

Patient: 뻣뻣해서 잘 움직이지 못하겠습니다.

Doctor: 통증은 간헐적인가요 아니면 항상 아픈가요?

Patient: 간헐적입니다.

Doctor: 통증이 다른 곳으로도 퍼지나요?

Patient: 예, 통증이 어깨 그리고 상완으로 퍼져요.

Doctor: 손목과 손에 저리거나 감각이 무뎌지는 것을 느끼십니까?

Patient: 네, 오른쪽 손목과 손에 저린 감각을 느낍니다.

Doctor: 전에도 이런 적이 있었나요?

Patient: 아니요.

Doctor: 알겠습니다. 제가 환자분의 목이 정상적인 선열을 가지고 있는지 검사하겠습니다. 또한 유연성도 확인하겠습니다. 제 지시사항을 따라주세요.

Patient: 알겠습니다.

3. 나의 통증이야기
독해구문

작열감

신체의 일부 또는 전체에 걸친 작열감은 결코 유쾌한 것은 아닙니다.

이것은 많은 기저질환들을 나타내는 징후가 되기도 합니다.

작열감과 동반하는 다른 증상에 따라, 원인이 심각한 외상 반응에서부터 혈관 질환 징후에 이르기까지 다양할 수도 있습니다.

허리에 눌리는 듯한 통증

나는 현재 부비동염으로 인해 항생제를 복용 중입니다. 그리고, 오른쪽 허리부분에 누르는 듯한 통증이 있습니다. 만일 신장염이 있는지 알기 위해 진료를 받으러 가야 하나요? 통증은 간헐적이며 결코 심하지는 않습니다. 나는 신장염과 관련된 그 밖의 증상들은 없습니다. 그러나, 통증 때문에 오른쪽으로 누울 수 없습니다. 그리고 때때로 이 통증을 왼쪽 부위에도 느끼지만 항상 허리부분에서 통증을 느낍니다.

당신의 조언에 감사드립니다.

잇몸이 창백하며 쓰라리고 아픕니다

나는 최근에 충치치료를 위해 치과에 갔습니다.

치과의사가 충치 치료를 한 후 그 치아는 매우 아프고 잇몸은 창백해졌고 아프며 쓰라립니다.

그 후 나는 다시 내원하여 그 이를 발치했습니다. 잇몸은 여전히 매우 창백하고 통증이 있고 쓰라립니다. 발치한 후 3주 이상이 되었습니다. 치아가 있었던 자리는 거의 치유가 되었습니다.

나의 질문은 왜 나의 잇몸이 이런 상태인가 입니다.

나의 남편은 여러 개의 치아를 발치했으나 이와 같은 것을 경험한 적이 결코 없었습니다. 이 일이 발생한지 6주 이상이 되었습니다.

4. 통증의 개념
해석

통증 (명사)

- 신체의 일부가 아플 때 느끼는 감각
그녀는 통증을 느껴요.

나의 통증이 심해져요.

나는 진통제를 복용하지 않았기에 통증이 심해졌어요.

통증이 점점 더 심해져요.

나는 만성 허리통증으로 시달립니다.

통증이 점점 잦아들고 있습니다.

통증이 멈췄습니다.

통증이 사라졌습니다.

아픈/통증이 느껴지는 (형용사)

-(정신적 육체적 모두) 통증을 느끼는

정신적으로:

그녀는 아버지의 죽음을 말하기에 여전히 고통스러워합니다.

육체적으로:

그는 아프고 부은 무릎관절을 호소합니다.

통증 (명사)

-지속적으로 아픈 통증

두통이 있어요.

배가 아파요

그녀는 이가 아파요.

통증을 느끼다 (동사)

- 지속적으로 통증을 느끼다.

온몸이 다 아팠어요.

나의 허리가 심하게 아팠어요.

나의 양쪽 발이 아팠어요.

여기저기 아픈 통증 (명사)

- 여기저기 동시다발로 아프지만 특별한 질병이 있는 것은 아님

많은 노인들은 여기저기가 아픈 통증으로 고생을 합니다.

쓰라림 (명사)

- 상처나 염증으로 인한 신체의 아프고 종종 빨간 부위

환자가 욕창이 생겼어요.

입술에 포진이 생겼어요.

통증 (명사)

- A pain or irritation 통증 또는 불편함

근육통은 새로운 운동프로그램을 시작하거나 현재 진행중인 운동프로그램을 변경하거나 또는 운동의 시간 또는 강도를 연장했을 때 느껴집니다.

쓰라린, 몸이 쑤시는 듯한 (형용사)

- 상처, 염증, 또는 과도한 운동으로 인한 통증의

인후염이 생겼어요.

두 발이 모두 아파요.

아프다 (동사)

- 신체적 정신적인 아픔을 모두 의미합니다.

통증을 느끼다.

신체의 일부를 아프게 하다.

정신적으로:

너의 말은 나에게 심한 상처를 줬어.

너의 감정을 상하게 하려는 의도는 아니었어.

신체적으로:

내 발목이 여전히 심하게 아프다.

다리가 너무 아파서 앉아야만 했다.

그녀는 넘어져서 다리를 약간 다쳤다.

달릴 때 무릎이 아파요.

4. 통증의 개념
연습문제 정답

1. A bee sting can be extremely *painful*.
2. She has a chest pain.
3. She completed the marathon and her body *ached* all over.
4. He made an appointment with the dentist because he couldn't put up with his *toothache* any longer.
5. I have an earache.
6. I was badly *hurt* in the accident.
7. She is suffering from chronic back *pain*.
8. Gardening aggravates my *backache*.
9. That spot is very *sore*, doctor.
10. After I took the analgesic, the *pain* wore off.
11. I can't walk. My ankle *hurts*.
12. My grandmother usually suffers from a lot of *pains* and *aches*.
13. I am very *sore* because of all that exercise.
14. Despite all the chiropractic adjustments, my back still *hurts* me.
15. He has a sore throat.

5. 통증발생 시간
주요구문 해석

통증이 언제부터 시작되었나요?

Q1. 통증이 언제부터 시작되었지요?

A1. 어제 밤부터 시작되었습니다.

Q2. 두통이 언제부터 시작되었나요?

A2. 약 일 주 전부터 시작되었어요.

Q3. 통증이 언제 처음 시작되었나요?

A3. 약 2~3일 전에 알게 되었어요.

통증이 하루 중 특정한 시간대에 발생하나요?

Q1. 통증이 낮에 시작되나요 또는 밤에 시작되나요?

A1. 제 생각에 통증이 낮에 시작되는 것 같아요.

Q2. 두통이 하루 중 특정한 시간대에 시작되나요?

A2. 제 생각에는 두통이 이른 아침에 시작되는 것 같습니다.
아침에 일어날 때 통증을 느낍니다.

Q3. 항상 통증을 느끼나요 아니면 특정 시간에 통증을 느끼나요?

A3. 음, 낮에는 괜찮습니다. 하지만 밤에는 통증 때문에 자다가 깨어납니다.

아프신지 얼마나 되셨습니까?

Q1. 얼마나 오랫동안 흉통이 있었나요?

A1. 흉통이 생긴지 약 2개월 되었습니다.

Q2. 이가 얼마 동안 아프셨나요?

A2. 지난주부터 아팠어요.

Q3. 요통으로 고생 하신지 얼마나 되셨나요?

A3. 이번에 생긴 허리통증은 4주 이상 지속되고 있습니다.

Q4. 구내염이 생긴지 얼마나 되셨나요?

A4. 2-3일 정도요.

예전에도 이런 통증이 있었나요?

Q1. 전에도 이런 통증을 느끼셨나요?

A1. 아닙니다. 전에 이런 종류의 통증을 느낀 적이 없습니다. 내게 새로운 종류의 통증입니다.

Q2. 이전에도 요통이 있었나요?

A2. 예. 전에도 요통이 있었지만, 이번 경우는 다르고 통증도 더 심합니다.

Q3. 전에도 흉통이 있었다면, 이번 통증은 전과 유사한가요 아니면 다른가요?

A3. 음, 지난 여름에 느꼈던 흉통과 아주 흡사해요.

5. 통증발생시간
나의 통증 설명하기

무릎관절통증

Patient: 내 무릎관절이 너무 아픕니다.

Doctor: 통증을 처음 느낀 게 언제입니까?

Patient: 내가 2틀 전 계단을 올라갈 때 알게 되었어요.

Doctor: 통증을 경감시키기 위해 하실 수 있는 일이 있습니까?

Patient: 음, 아픈 부위를 높이 올리면 통증이 경감되는 것 같아요.

Doctor: 통증이 사라지는데 얼마나 걸리나요?

Patient: 하루 정도 걸립니다.

Doctor: 무릎을 검사하겠으니 침대에 올라오셔서 등을 대고 누우시겠습니까?

Patient: 알겠습니다.

Doctor: 무릎을 굽히겠습니다. 느낌이 어떤가요?

Patient: 너무 아파요.

6. 통증의 강도
주요구문 해석

통증이 얼마나 심한가요?

Q1. 통증이 얼마나 심한가요?/통증이 얼마나 심한지 말씀해 주시겠습니까?

A1. 아주 심합니다. 무릎관절이 칼로 찌르는 듯이 아파요.

Q2. 두통으로 인해 잠에서 깬 적이 있습니까?

A2. 예. 심한 두통으로 인해 밤에 잘 수가 없습니다.

Q3. 통증이 너무 심해서 밤에 잠을 잘 수가 없나요?

A3. 예. 허리가 너무 아파서 밤새 엎치락뒤치락 해요.

6. 통증의 강도
나의 통증 설명하기

흉통

Doctor: 어디가 아프십니까?

Patient: 음, 가슴과 팔에 통증을 느끼고 손가락은 저릿저릿 합니다.

Doctor: 알겠습니다. 언제 통증을 처음 느끼셨습니까?

Patient: 음, 약 한달 전쯤이라고 생각됩니다.

Doctor: 통증을 "경미한, 보통의, 심한 또는 아주 심한" 이란 단어를 사용하여 표현해 주시겠습니까?

Patient: 심한 통증입니다.

Doctor: 알겠습니다. 통증이 언제 처음 시작되었는지 기억나십니까?

Patient: 네. 조깅할 때 심한 통증을 느꼈습니다. 통증이 너무 심해서 숨을 쉴 수조차도 없었습니다.

Doctor: 통증은 얼마나 오랫동안 지속되었나요?

Patient: 음. 대략 십분 정도 였습니다.

Doctor: 알겠습니다. 심장소리를 들어보겠습니다. 셔츠를 올려주세요.

7. 통증척도표 0-10

통증척도표의 역사

눈으로 말하는 위대한 대화법-“얼마나 아프세요”

이 통증척도표는 80년대 초반 간호사인 Donna Wong 과 소아과 전문의인 Connie Morain Baker 두 분이 통증을 표현하기 어려운 어린 환자들, 특히 그 중에서도 화상을 입은 어린이들을 돕기 위해 고안한 것입니다.

이 두 분은 50명 이상의 어린 환자에게 "통증이 없을 때"부터 “가장 아픈 때”를 나타내는 얼굴을 그려보라 고 했습니다.

어린 환자들은 그 당시 인기 있던 "웃는 모습의 스티커" (🙂)를 출발점으로 사용했습니다. Wong과 Baker는 어린 환자들이 그린 이처럼 다양한 얼굴 표정의 그림을 받았습니다.

후에 한 화가는 이 통증척도표에 맞게 얼굴의 표정들을 더 간소화 하였습니다. 이 화가는 얼굴의 눈썹부분을 좀 더 다양화한 것을 제외하고는 어린 환자들이 그린 얼굴 표정을 통증표에 적용하였습니다.

7. 통증척도표 0-10

통증척도표 만들기

정답

0 	1-2	3 	4	5 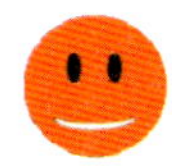
No Pain	Tender Blunt	Manageable	Dull Nagging	Aching

6	7 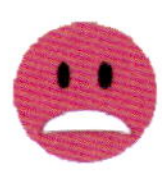	8	9 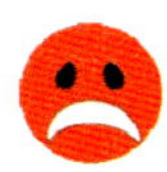	10 **The worst possible**
Gnawing Throbbing	Gripping	Horrible	Unbearable distress	Agonizing Excruciating

7. 통증척도표 0-10 주요구문 해석

통증척도표 0-10을 사용한다면, 통증이 몇 점 정도인가요?

Q1. 통증척도표 1-10을 사용한다면, 지금 몇 점 정도의 통증을 느끼나요?

A1. 나의 통증은 8점 정도이며 항상 통증이 있습니다. 통증이 없다는 것이 어떠한지 더 이상 잘 모르겠습니다. 지난 10년 동안 이러했습니다.

Q2. 오늘은 통증을 얼마나 느끼십니까?

A2. 약 11점입니다. 아파서 죽을 것만 같아요.

Q3. 1점이 가장 적은 통증이고 10점이 가장 큰 통증인 통증척도표 1-10에서 환자분의 통증수치는 몇 점 정도입니까?

A3. 나는 통증을 느끼는 최고치가 상당히 높은 편이지만, 통증이 9.5점 정도가 되는 것 같습니다.

7. 통증척도표 0-10
나의 통증 설명하기

치통

Doctor: 치통이 시작되면 얼마나 오랫동안 지속되나요?

Patient: 주로 30분 정도 지속됩니다.

Doctor: 언제 처음 알게 되었지요?

Patient: 음. 내 어금니 중 하나가 아픈 것을 나흘 전에 알게 되었어요.

Doctor: 어떤 통증인지 설명해 주시겠어요?

Patient: 칼로 찌르는 듯한 심한 통증입니다.

Doctor: 만일 통증을 1-10으로 표현한다면, 몇 점 정도 일까요?

Patient: 만약 1000이 통증척도표에 있었다면 아마 1000점 정도요.

Doctor: 오! 무엇이 통증을 악화시키나요?

Patient: 단 음식을 먹은 후에 이가 더 아파져요.

Doctor: 우선, 충치가 있는지 확인하기 위해 엑스레이를 찍겠습니다.

8. 통증의 기간
주요구문 해석

통증이 지속적인가요 또는 간헐적인가요?

Q1. 통증이 시작될 때 갑작스럽게 아팠나요 아니면 서서히 아픈가요?
A1. 예기치 못하게 갑작스럽게 아프기 시작했어요.

Q2. 목의 통증이 지속적인가요 아니면 간헐적인가요?
A2. 간헐적입니다./음, 항상 통증을 느낍니다. 3년 이상 이 통증이 계속되고 있습니다.

Q3. 통증이 갑자기 시작됐나요?
A3. 예. 갑자기 아주 심하게 통증이 시작됐습니다.

8. 통증의 기간
나의 통증 설명하기

계절성 엘러지

Doctor: 계절성 앨러지와 수반되는 다른 증상이 있습니까?

Patient: 예. 편두통이 있어요.

Doctor: 당신의 편두통이 어떤지 설명해 주시겠습니까?

Patient: 음, 찌르는 듯한 예리한 통증입니다.

Doctor: 머리의 어느 부위가 가장 아프십니까?

Patient: 왼쪽 관자놀이가 몹시 아픕니다.

Doctor: 편두통이 시작될 때 수반되었던 다른 증상을 말씀해 주시겠습니까?

Patient: 음, 양쪽 눈이 거의 한 시간 동안 흐릿하게 보여요.

Doctor: 편두통이 간헐적인가요 또는 지속적인가요?

Patient: 간헐적입니다.

Doctor: 편두통이 하루 중 특정한 시간대에 악화되나요?

Patient: 예. 아침이면 특히 악화됩니다.

9. 통증을 야기시키는 원인
주요구문 해석

통증이 처음 시작될 때 무엇을 하고 계셨나요?

Q1. 통증이 시작될 때 무엇을 하고 계셨나요?

A1. 계단을 오르고 있었어요.

Q2. 요통이 시작될 때 무엇을 하고 계셨나요?

A2. 쓰레기를 버리고 있었습니다.

Q3. 통증이 시작되기 전에 무엇을 하고 계셨나요?

A3. 무거운 것을 들고 있었습니다.

통증을 야기시키는 특별한 것이 있나요?

Q1. 무엇이 통증을 야기시키나요?

A1. 무엇이 통증을 야기시키는지 모르겠습니다.

Q2. 통증을 야기시키는 음식이 있나요?

A2. 내 생각에는 적포도주를 마실 때마다 편두통이 오는 것 같아요.

Q3. 군집성 두통을 야기시키는 음식이 있나요?

A3. 음, 내가 카페인이 든 음료를 섭취할 때마다 두통이 발생되는 것 같아요.

9. 통증을 야기시키는 원인
나의 통증 설명하기

속쓰림

Doctor: 스미스 선생님 나는 국제진료소의 의사입니다. 어디가 아프십니까?

Mr. Smith: 배가 심하게 아파요.

Doctor: 어떻게 아프신지 설명해 주시겠습니까?

Mr. Smith: 음, 배 윗부분을 칼로 찌르는 듯한 통증입니다.

Doctor: 위를 자극할 만한 음식을 드셨나요?

Mr. Jung: 사실, 어젯밤에 맥주를 마셨습니다. 하지만 조금만 마셨습니다..

Doctor: 통증을 악화시키는 것이 있습니까?

Mr. Smith: 제 생각에는 제가 매운 음식을 먹을 때마다 위가 아파요.

Doctor: 복부를 검사하겠습니다. 그러기 위해서는 여기 검사대에 누우셔야 합니다. 제가 도와드리겠습니다.

Mr. Smith: 감사합니다.

Doctor: 천만에요. 편안하십니까?

Mr. Smith: 예.

Chapter 5

Doctor: 복부청진을 하겠습니다. 가운을 올려주시겠습니까?

Mr. Smith: 이렇게요?

Doctor: 예. 스미스 선생님, 이제 복부를 살짝 누른 후 세게 누르겠습니다. 눌렀을 때 아프거나 불편함을 느끼시면 말씀해 주세요.

Mr. Smith: 아야. 오른쪽 배요. 정말 아픕니다.

Doctor: 죄송합니다. 이제 꾸욱 눌렀다가 떼겠습니다. 꾸욱 눌렀을 때 아픈지 아니면 떼었을 때 아픈지 말씀해 주세요.

Mr. Smith: 알겠습니다.

Doctor: 마지막으로 복부의 여러 부위를 두드리겠습니다. 만일 아프시면 말씀하세요.

Mr. Smith: 알겠습니다.

10. 통증의 완화 및 악화
주요구문

무엇이 통증을 완화 시키나요?

Q1. 진통제를 복용하면 관절통증이 완화되나요?

A1. 예. 진통제를 복용하면, 관절통증이 멈춥니다

Q2. 통증을 완화시키는 것이 있습니까?

A2. 예. 만일 내가 한참 동안 앉거나 누워있으면, 훨씬 더 나아져요. 또한 앉은 자세에서 서있는 자세로 바꾸면 통증이 완화 되요.

Q3. 온 찜질이나 냉 찜질을 하면, 통증완화에 도움이 되나요?

A3. 예. 온 찜질이 특히 좋아요.

무엇이 통증을 악화시키나요?

Q1. 통증을 악화시키는 것이 있습니까?

A1. 예. 만일 같은 자세로 오래 앉아있거나 서 있으면 허리와 엉덩이 부위에 심한 통증을 느낍니다.

Q2. 커피가 두통을 악화시키나요?

A2. 아니요.

Q3. 무엇이 통증을 악화시키나요?

A3. 비가 오거나 날씨가 추워지면 통증이 더 심해집니다. 설상가상으로 그런 날에는 진통제도 거의 듣지 않습니다.

통증이 점점 완화 또는 악화 되나요?

Q1. 통증이 시간이 지나면서 계속 더 악화가 됐나요, 아니면 거의 같은 정도 인가요?

A1. 사실, 지난 두 주간 점차적으로 악화되고 있습니다.

Q2. 두통이 점점 더 심해지나요?

A2. 예. 점점 심해져요.

Q3. 통증이 하루 중 특별한 시간대에 더 악화되나요?

A3. 예. 계속 통증을 느끼지만, 밤이 되면 더 심하게 아파져요.

10. 통증의 완화 및 악화
나의 통증 설명하기

군집성 두통

Dr. Park: 차트에 심한 두통이 있다고 적혀 있군요. 그럼 두통을 설명해 주시겠습니까? 어떤 통증입니까?

Mr. Jung: 예리한 것으로 찌르는 듯하며 참을 수 없을 정도로 심합니다.

Dr. Park: 알겠습니다. 1점은 가장 통증이 약하고 10점이 통증이 가장 심한 1~10의 통증척도표를 사용한다면, 현재 통증이 몇 점 정도가 될까요?

Mr. Jung: 9점 정도요. 지난 3-4일 동안 내가 겪은 통증은 평생에서 겪어 본 가장 심한 통증이었습니다. 아주 끔찍 했습니다.

Dr. Park: 통증이 보통 얼마나 지속되나요?

Mr. Jung: 음. 일정하지는 않아요. 주로 하루 동안 아프지만 오후에는 통증이 잦아듭니다. 그러나 지난주에는 통증이 너무 심해서 전혀 거동을 할 수가 없었어요.

Dr. Park: 알겠습니다. 주로 어느 부위가 아픈가요?

Mr. Jung: 머리 오른쪽 부분이 주로 아파요. 하지만 결코 머리 양쪽 부분이 모두 아프지는 않아요.

Dr. Park: 통증이 다른 곳으로도 옮겨가나요?

Mr. Jung: 그렇지는 않습니다. 하지만 같은 쪽의 눈과 뺨에 통증을 느낍니다.

Dr. Park: 머리 오른쪽 부위만 아프고 같은 쪽의 눈 주위와 뺨이 아프다고 했지요, 그렇지요?

Mr. Jung: 맞습니다.

Dr. Park: 아픈 부위를 손가락으로 가리켜 주시겠습니까?

Mr. Jung: 바로 여기요...그리고 여기도요.

Dr. Park: 어느 부위인지 알겠습니다. 통증은 주로 머리 앞부분이고, 이마, 오른쪽 관자놀이, 눈과 뺨 부분이군요.

Mr. Jung: 그렇습니다. 다행히도 머리 뒷 부분은 아프지 않습니다.

Dr. Park: 통증을 야기시키는 음식이 있습니까?

제 말은 두통을 일으키는 특정 음식이 있느냐는 것입니다.

Mr. Jung: 음. 제 생각에는 커피와 같이 카페인이 들어 있는 음료를 마실 때 두통이 생기는 것 같습니다.

Dr. Park: 커피요! 그러면 아플 때 통증을 완화시켜주는 것이 있습니까?

Mr. Jung: 없습니다. 아주 강력한 진통제도 제 두통엔 잘 듣지 않습니다. 제가 왜 이런 통증이 있나요?

Dr. Park: 제 소견에 의하면 정 선생님은 군집성 두통을 앓고 있습니다. 군집성 두통은 0대의 남성에게서 주로 나타나며 머리의 오른쪽 또는 왼쪽 부분에만 통증이 나타납니다. 환자분은 우선 카페인이든 음료를 금해야 합니다. 왜냐하면 환자분의 두통을 야기시키는 요소들 중 하나가 카페인이든 음료이기 때문입니다.

Mr. Jung: 그러면, 커피와 다른 카페인이 들어있는 음료를 마시지 않겠습니다.

11. 통증일지 작성법
정답

통증일지 작성법							
날짜	통증이 언제부터 시작되었나요?	어디가 아픈가요?	무엇을 하던 중이었나요?	어떠한 통증인가요?	통증이 얼마나 심한가요? 통증척도표 0-10을 사용하세요	통증이 얼마나 오래 동안 지속되었나요?	호전되기 위해서 무엇을 하셨나요?
6월 16일	아침 늦게	허리에	운동 중	날카롭게 느껴지는 통증	8	30분	약을 복용하고 휴식을 취했음
6월 17일	자정 무렵	왼쪽 관자놀이	잠을 청하려는 도중	욱신거리는	3	약 2시간 정도	진통제를 복용하였음
6월 18일	Right before the sleep	Calf	Trying to sleep	Sore	5	Persistent	Applied thin coat of leg lifting cream then rubbed it
6월 19일	Early in the morning	Front part of my head	After drinking a cup of coffee	Throbbing	6	About 3 hours	Took a pain killer

Chapter 6
Directions for Taking Medications
복약지시

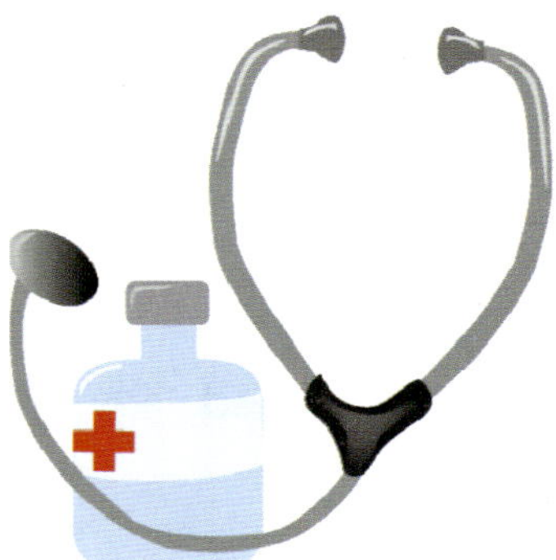

1. Medications
약

- **Key Words, 주요어휘**

  A. Pharmacy Related Words, 약국과 관련된 어휘

  - Quiz: 내 단어장 점검하기
  - Drill: Word Search Puzzle, 연습문제: 어휘퍼즐

  B. Types of Medication, 약의 종류

  - Quiz: 내 단어장 점검하기
  - Drill: Word Search Puzzle, 연습문제: 어휘퍼즐

  C. Names of Medication, 약의 이름

  - Quiz: 내 단어장 점검하기
  - Drill, 연습문제
  - Words, 어휘

- **Getting My Prescription Filled, 약 처방 받기**
  - Dialogue, 대화
  - Words, 어휘
  - Review, 복습

- **Words Review, 어휘복습**

Key Words

A. Pharmacy Related Words

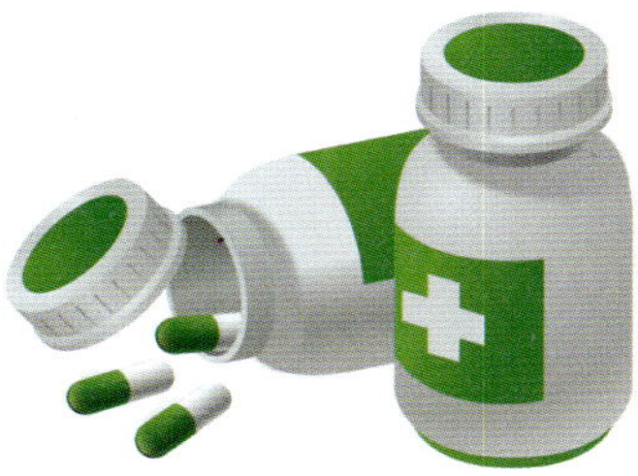

Prescription: 처방전

Prescription Medicine: 처방전이 필요한 약

Over-the-counter (OTC) Medicine: 처방전 없이 구할 수 있는 약

Generic drug: 카피약(복제의약품)

Brand name drug: 오리지널 의약품

Pharmacist: 약사

Pharmacy/A drugstore: 약국

Inactive ingredient like things in the drug, such as colors or flavorings: 색소(식염) 또는 맛을 내는 첨가물과 같은 약효와 상관없는 성분

Allergic reaction: 과민반응

Therapeutic (having the ability to heal): 치료상의

Side effects: 부작용

Drowsy/Sleepy: 졸린

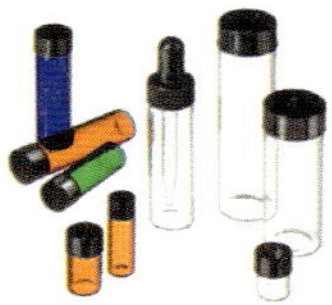

Medication vials: 약병

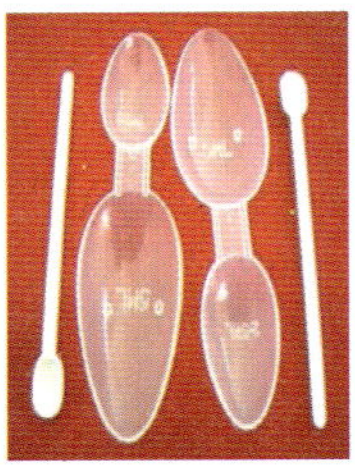

Dose-measuring spoon: 복용량 측정 스푼

Grain spoon: 가루약 스푼

Dose: 복용량

Overdose: 과다복용

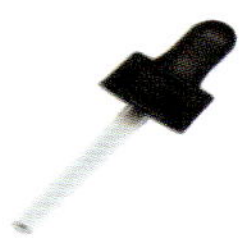

Eye-dropper: 점안기/점적기

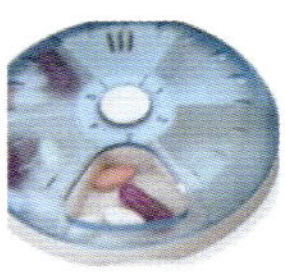

Pill-box: 약 담는 용기

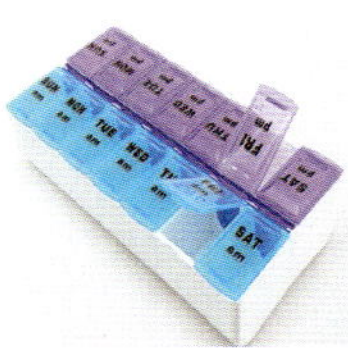

7-Day Pill-Box/7-Day Pill Organizer for weekly course of medication: 일주일 복용 분량의 약을 담는 통

QUIZ: 내 단어장 점검하기 !!

아래 단어 및 구문을 읽고 알맞은 어휘를 적으세요.

Prescription: ....

Prescription Medicine: ....

Pharmacist: ....

Generic drug: ....

Allergic reaction: ....

Grain spoon: ....

Medication vials: ....

Brand name drug: ....

Overdose: ....

Eye-dropper: ....

Therapeutic (having the ability to heal): ....

Drowsy/Sleepy: ....

Over-the-counter (OTC) Medicine: ....

Side effects: ....

7-Day Pill-Box/7-Day Pill Organizer for weekly course of medication : ....

Drill: 아래의 단어를 Word Search Puzzle에서 찾아보세요.

M	C	G	X	O	I	A	E	K	S	O	T	D	E	G	X	M
T	M	E	T	D	R	L	P	X	X	N	Q	T	Y	U	B	U
P	B	N	W	Q	L	L	V	L	N	B	F	Q	C	R	L	E
T	H	E	R	A	P	E	U	T	I	C	K	C	A	M	Y	S
X	P	R	E	S	C	R	I	P	T	I	O	N	J	E	G	O
G	X	I	H	D	F	G	S	A	D	H	D	U	D	I	X	Y
S	M	C	Y	K	L	I	N	B	N		N	R	K	H	Q	N
U	D		O	N	L	C	M	Q	N	T	O	I	E	J	X	Q
J	B	D	H	E	R		F	A	O	P	R	C	I	U	U	J
E	E	R	B	R	Y	R	M	U	P	O	E	P	Q	Y	B	G
E	S	U	S	I	D	E		E	F	F	E	C	T	S	G	H
A	U	G	F	P		A	R	O	N	L	J	Q	R	D	O	Y
D	G	M	E	D	I	C	A	T	I	O	N		V	I	A	L
J	D	I	R	N	W	T	Y	E	J	N	G	L	K	H	Q	T
S	J	U	B	K	U	I	S	O	V	O	K	H	O	C	C	F
A	G	L	F	P	O	O	V	E	R	D	O	S	E	G	A	V
M	G	G	R	A	I	N		S	P	O	O	N	D	B	C	M

처방전, 카피약, 오리지널 의약품, 과민반응, 치료상의, 약병,

가루약 스푼, 과다복용, 점안기/점적기, 부작용

B. Types of Medication

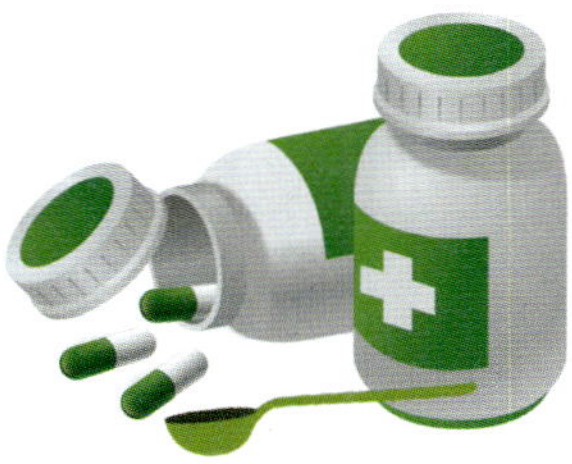

Stool softener: 변 연화제

Suppository: 좌약

Enema solution: 관장약

Bottle of cough syrup: 감기약(물약)

Antipyretic medication: 해열제

Antitussives: 진해제

Ointment: 연고

Liquid medication: 물약

Steroid cream: 스테로이드 연고

Steroid free cream: 스테로이드를 첨가하지 않은 연고

Herb medication: 한약

Natural medication: 생약

Eye drops: 점안액

Lozenge: 목 캔디와 같은 빨아먹는 약

Transdermal patch: 피부접착제 패취

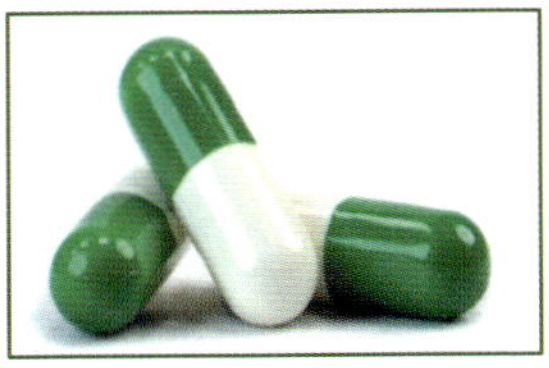

Capsule: 캡슐

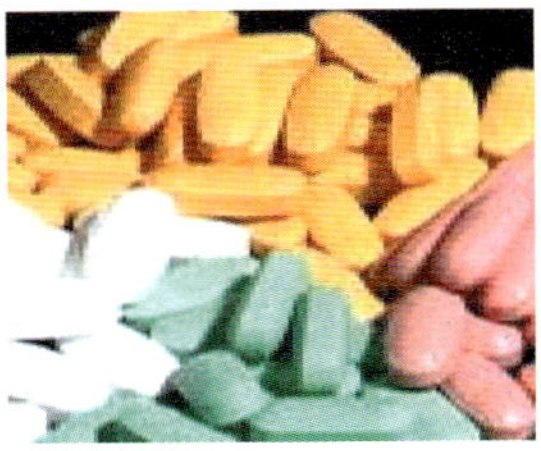

Tablet: 알약

* Tablet의 모양은 다양함

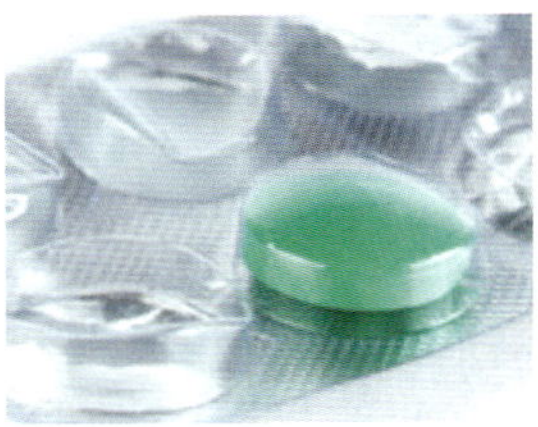

Pill (Anything small and round for a specific dose of medicine**):** 알약(작고 둥근 알약)

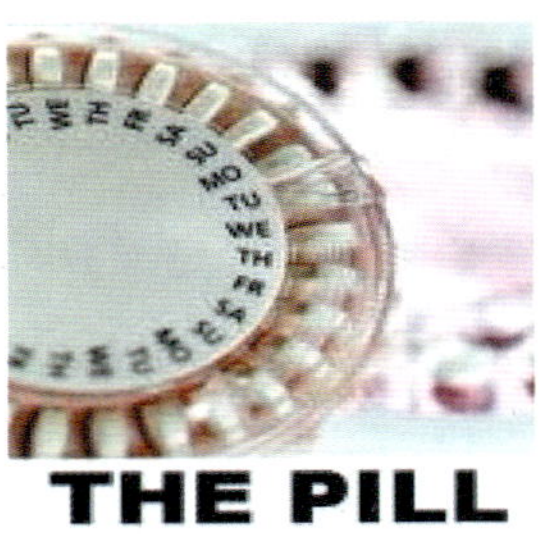

The Pill (A general nickname for the combinec oral contraceptive pill**):** 피임약(경구피임약의 애칭)

QUIZ: 내 단어장 점검하기 !!

아래 단어 및 구문을 읽고 알맞은 어휘를 적으세요.

The Pill: ....

Tablet: ....

Transdermal patch: ....

Lozenge: ....

Herbal medication: ....

Antitussives: ....

Ointment: ....

Antipyretic medication: ....

Stool softener: ....

Suppository: ....

Enema solution: ....

Bottle of cough syrup: ....

Liquid medication: ....

Pill: ....

Eye drops: ....

Steroid free cream: ....

Drill: 아래의 단어를 Word Search Puzzle에서 찾아 보세요.

X	X	S	N	Y	S	O	I	N	T	M	E	N	T	L	G	I	W
K	W	Q	A	P	M	N	N	Q	R	U	E	B	M	S	M	L	B
I	K	Q	T	F	G	O	M	A	A	V	O	J	J	B	I	C	A
W	A	C	U	T	H	C	F	W	N	X	K	C	Y	Q	J	W	S
J	B	U	R	L	R	D	E	C	S	R	T	C	U	H	L	M	Q
X	B	J	A	F	M	S	J	Y	D	M	S	I	K	X	L	M	L
D	P	X	L	V	M	U	O	B	E	V	D	P	B	F	C	F	I
L	V	P		J	L	P	H	B	R		V	L	S	J	X	H	T
E	X	B	M	R	D	P	V	N	M	M	D	A	A	E	B	F	Y
E	I	Q	E	A	M	O	H	E	A	E	R	R	W	K	M	V	U
P	U	O	D	L	L	S	D	E	L	K	X	I	O	A	U	I	C
I	M	I	I	P	J	I	X	L		N	M	G	S	P	X	X	H
T	C	I	C	H	C	T	B	D	P	N	X	O	H	B	S	Y	F
K	K	F	A	A	Y	O	J	C	A	C	L	M	N	N	E	I	N
E	D	Q	T	X	K	R	T	G	T	Q	N	G	D	U	P	M	P
E	B	I	I	B	A	Y	P	Y	C	A	O	L	C	U	U	X	K
N	O	L	O	Z	E	N	G	E	H	U	X	G	W	I	O	F	P
N	M	A	N	T	I	T	U	S	S	I	V	E	S	U	L	N	F

좌약, 진해제, 연고, 물약, 생약, 점안액,

목캔디와 같은 빨아먹는 약, 피부접착제 패취

C. Names of Medication

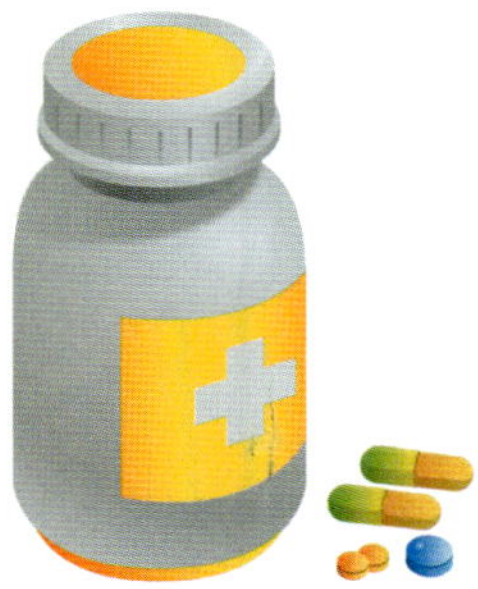

Mosquito repellent: 모기퇴치제

Mosquito coils: 모기향

Mosquito repellent bracelet: 모기퇴치제 팔찌

Lubricant eye drops/Dry eye relief/Artificial tears: 인공눈물

Redness relief lubricant/Redness reliever eye drops: 충혈 제거 안약

Eye allergy relief drops: 앨러지 안약

Disinfectant/Antiseptics (A topical antiseptic): 소독약(외상에 바르는 소독약)

Bandage/Band-aid: 일회용 반창고/반창고 제품명

Throat lozenge: 목 캔디

Laxative: 변비약

Hemorrhoid relief cream: 치질 연고

Iron: 철분약

Contraceptive pill: 피임약

Antacid: 제산제

Antibiotics: 항생제

Chapter 6

Anti-inflammatory: 소염제

Antidepressant: 항우울제

Sedative: 안정제

Diuretic/Water pill: 이뇨제

Motion sickness relief medication: 멀미약

Sleeping pill/Sleeping aid: 수면제

Pain reliever/Pain killer/Pain control medication: 진통제

Bronchodilator: 기관지 확장제

Nebulizer: 네블라이져

Fever reducer: 해열제

Cough suppressant: 기침 억제제(진해제)

Expectorant: 거담제

Nicotine patch: 금연 패취

Back patch: 등, 허리에 부치는 파스

QUIZ: 내 단어장 점검하기 !!

아래 단어 및 구문을 읽고 알맞은 어휘를 적으세요.

Mosquito coils: ....

Throat lozenge: ....

Laxative: ....

Iron: ....

Contraceptive pill: ....

Antacid: ....

Hemorrhoid relief cream: ....

Antibiotics: ....

Anti-inflammatory: ....

Back patch: ....

Expectorant: ....

Cough suppressant: ....

Fever reducer: ....

Nicotine patch: ....

Antidepressant: ....

Sleeping pill/Sleeping aid: ....

Diuretic/Water pill: ....

Motion sickness relief medication: ....

Redness reliever eye drops: ....

Mosquito repellent: ....

Mosquito repellent bracelet: ....

Antiseptics: ....

Artificial tears: ....

Dry eye relief: ....

Eye allergy relief drops: ....

Disinfectant: ....

Sedative: ....

Redness relief lubricant: ....

Bronchodilator: ....

Pain control medication: ....

Nebulizer: ....

Pain reliever: ....

Drill: 각각의 약 이름을 영어와 한국말로 적으세요.

정답은 페이지301을 참고하세요.

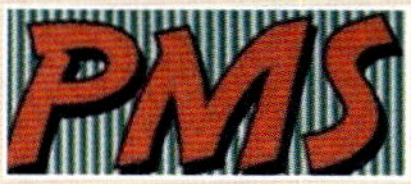

Eliminate water weight due to premenstrual and menstrual bloat, water gain & puffiness

1. (   )

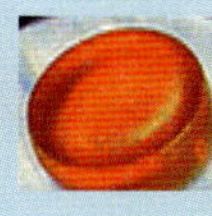

Fast acting
Sore throat relief

2. (   )

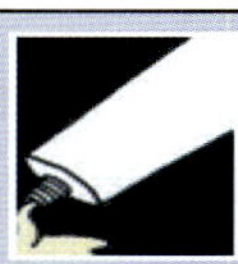

Temporarily provides a coating for relief of anorectal discomforts

3. (   )

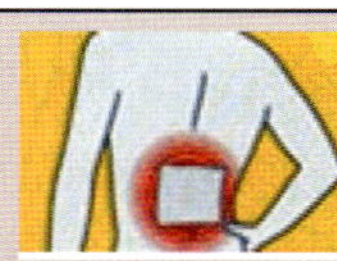

Simple backache, arthritis, strains, bruises, spasm

4. (   )

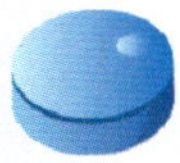

To help reduce difficulty in falling asleep

5. (   )

Fast effective relief from acid indigestion and heartburn

6. (   )

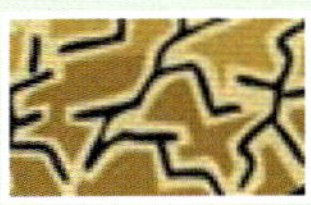

Relieves LASIK dryness
Relief with every blink

7. (   )

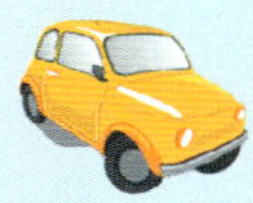

Prevent nausea, dizziness & vomiting.
Dosage should be taken one hour before travel starts.
All day relief

8. (   )

Words

eliminate water: 몸에 과다 축적된 수분을 제거

premenstrual and menstrual bloat: 생리전과 생리 중 아랫배의 팽만감

water gain: 수분축적으로 인해 부은

puffiness: 푸석푸석하게 부은

fast acting: 효과 빠른

sore throat relief: 인후염의 완화

anorectal discomforts: 항문과 직장부위의 통증

backache: 허리통증

arthritis: 관절염

strains: (발목을) 삐다. 염좌

bruises: 타박상

spasm: 근육경련

acid indigestion: 위산과다로 인한 소화불량

heartburn: 속쓰림

LASIK dryness: LASIK 수술과 관련된 안구 건조증

nausea: 오심, 메스꺼움

dizziness: 어지러움증

vomiting: 구토

all day relief: 24시간 동안 약효가 계속 지속되는

Getting My Prescription Filled

At the local pharmacy in America

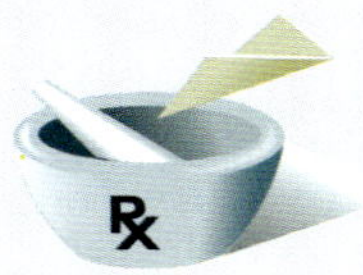

Pharmacist: Good morning. May I help you?

Mr. Smith: Yes. I need to get my prescription filled.

Pharmacist: Alright. Can I see your prescription slip?

Mr. Smith: Sure. Here it is. Well, I also need a dental floss and a chap stick. Where are those?

Pharmacist: The dental floss is on aisle 4, on the middle shelf and chap sticks are on aisle 3, on the top shelf.

Mr. Smith: Thanks.

Pharmacist: Will that be all?

Mr. Smith: That should do it.

Pharmacist: The total comes to $20.50.

Mr. Smith: That's a lot cheaper than the last one.

Pharmacist: Well, your prescription is brand name medication. It is quite expensive. Thus you have asked your doctor for me to get you a generic medication. So the price is a lot cheaper this time. As you know the generic drug is about half that price.

Mr. Smith: I see.

Pharmacist: Here's your medication. Have a good day.

Mr. Smith: You, too. Thank you.

Words

prescription slip: 처방전(용지)

generic drug: 카피약(복제의약품)

brand name medication: 오리지널 약

dental floss: 치실

chap stick: 챕스틱(입술 튼데 바르는 것)

Will that be all? 더 필요한 것이 있습니까?

half that price: 가격의 반액

Review: 각각의 구문을 영작하세요.
정답은 전 페이지의 Dialogue를 참고하세요.

Pharmacist: Good morning. May I help you?

Mr. Smith: 예. 처방전대로 약을 지어주세요.

Pharmacist: 알겠습니다. 처방전을 보여 주세요.

Mr. Smith: Sure. Here it is.

음. 그리고 치실과 챕스틱도 필요합니다.

Where are those?

Pharmacist: 치실은 4번 통로 중간 선반 위에 있고, 챕스틱은 3번 통로 맨 위의 선반 위에 있습니다.

Mr. Smith: Thanks.

Pharmacist: 더 필요한 것이 있습니까?

Mr. Smith: That should do it.

Pharmacist: 다 합해서 $20.50입니다.

Mr. Smith: That's a lot cheaper than the last one.

Pharmacist: 음, 고객님이 처방 받은 약은 오리지널 약입니다.

오리지널 약은 상당히 비쌉니다.

그래서 고객님이 의사에게 카피약으로 처방해달라고 요청하셔서 이번에 가격이 더 저렴합니다.

아시다시피 카피약은 오리지널 약 가격의 반액이기 때문입니다.

Mr. Smith: I see.

Pharmacist: Here's your medication. Have a good day.
Mr. Smith: You, too. Thank you.

Word Review: 위의 단어들을 복습하는 공간입니다.
정답은 Key Words를 참고하세요.

뜻: In English

처방전: ______________________________

처방전이 필요한 약: ______________________________

처방전 없이 구할 수 있는 약: ______________________________

카피약(복제의약품): ______________________________

오리지널 의약품: ______________________________

약사: ______________________________

과다복용: ______________________________

약국: ______________________________

과민반응: ______________________________

치료상의: ______________________________

부작용: ______________________________

졸린: ______________________________

일주일 복용 분량의 약을 담는 통: ______________________________

약병: ______________________________

복용량:____

약 담는 용기:____________________________________

점안기/점적기:___________________________________

복용량 측정 스푼:________________________________

가루약 스푼:_____________________________________

변 연화제:_______________________________________

좌약:____

관장약:____

감기약(물약):____________________________________

해열제:____

진해제:____

연고:____

물약:____

스테로이드 연고:_________________________________

스테로이드를 첨가하지 않은 연고:__________________

생약:____

한약:____

색소(식염) 또는 맛을 내는 첨가물과 같은 약효와 상관없는 성분:__________

____

점안액:________________

목 캔디와 같은 빨아먹는 약:________________

피부접착제 패취:________________

캡슐:________________

알약:________________

알약(작고 둥근 알약):________________

피임약(경구피임약의 애칭):________________

모기퇴치제:________________

모기향:________________

안정제:________________

소염제:________________

피임약:________________

제산제:________________

항생제:________________

항우울제:________________

목 캔디:________________

철분약:________________

일회용 반창고:________________

변비약:____________________

모기퇴치제 팔찌:____________________

인공눈물:____________________

소독약:____________________

충혈 제거 안약:____________________

치질 연고:____________________

앨러지 안약:____________________

이뇨제:____________________

멀미약:____________________

수면제:____________________

진통제:____________________

기관지 확장제:____________________

네블라이져:____________________

해열제:____________________

기침 억제제(진해제):____________________

거담제:____________________

금연 패취:____________________

등, 허리에 부치는 파스:____________________

2. Prescription 처방전

- **What does RX mean?**
  - **Code Breaker's Corner: 로리와 함께하는 미국문화 엿보기**
  - Doctor's handwriting, 의사의 자필로 쓴 처방전
  - What does the cartoon say?, 삽화가 뜻하는 의미는?
  - Words, 어휘
- **Prescription Slip in America, 미국처방전**
  - Sample Prescription, 처방전 샘플
  - What does the prescription say?, 처방전에 무엇이 적혀있나요?
  - Words, 어휘
  - Drill: Abbreviations, 연습문제: 약어
  - Drill: How to read a prescription slip, 연습문제: 처방전 읽는 방법
- **Reading Material, 독해구문**
  - Prescription Bottle, 처방전 약을 담은 용기
  - What's on the prescription bottle label?, 처방전 약병의 라벨에 무엇이 기재되어 있나요?
  - Words, 어휘

· Getting My Prescription Filled, 약 처방 받기

- Dialogue, 대화
- Words, 어휘
- Review, 복습

What does RX mean?

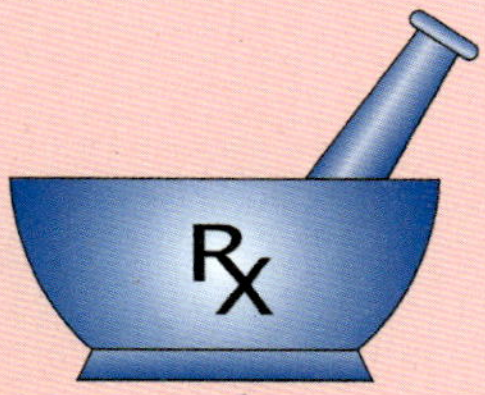

Some people think that Rx means prescription.

In a way it does.

However, Rx is the abbreviation for the Latin word meaning "recipe".

Code Breaker's Corner: 로리와 함께하는 미국문화 엿보기

Doctor's handwriting

미국의 처방전은 의사가 자필로 씁니다. 자필을 잘 알아볼 수 없을 정도의 악필이 종종 있기 때문에 약사들이 처방전의 필체를 읽을 수 없어 약을 조제할 때 어려움을 겪기도 합니다.

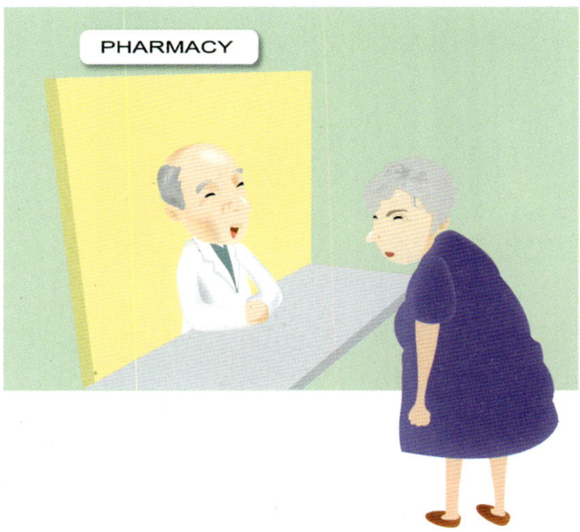

"I had trouble reading your doctor's handwriting, but I think I finally figured it out. However, if you start to drool uncontrollably or gain more than 20 pounds in 10 days, stop taking these medications immediately"

What does the cartoon say?

"I had trouble reading your doctor's handwriting, but I think I finally figured it out. However, if you start to drool uncontrollably or gain more than 20 pounds in 10 days, stop taking these medications immediately"

Words

handwriting: 필체

drool: 침을 질질 흘리다

uncontrollably: 주체할 수 없이

gain: 체중이 늘다

immediately: 즉시

Prescription Slip in America

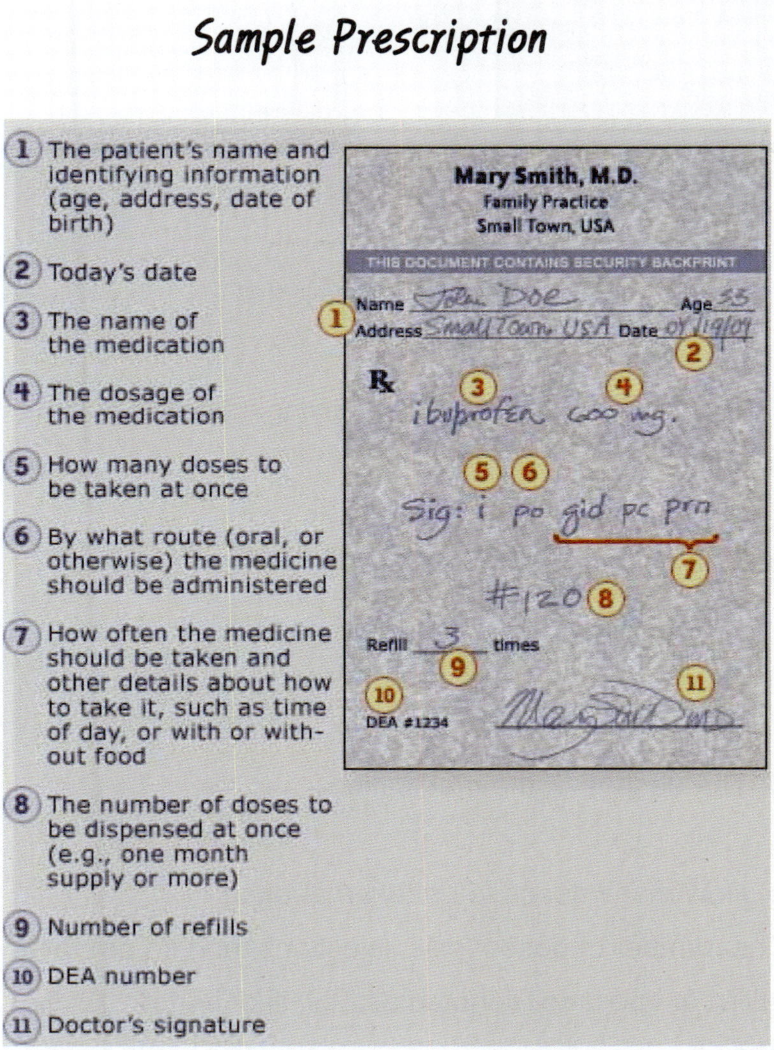

Source: http://www.intelihealth.com

다음 페이지에 위의 Sample Prescription을 다시 적음

What does ths prescription say?

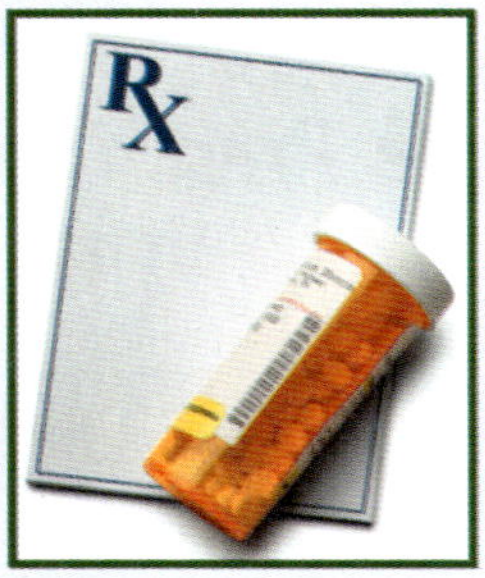

(위의 처방전을 다시 적음)

1. The patient's name and identifying information (age, address, date of birth)

2. Today's date

3. The name of the medication

4. The dosage of the medication

5. How many doses to be taken at once:
The number of doses (pills, injections, and so on) to be taken at one time, denoted as "i, ii, iii or iv" for 1, 2, 3 or 4; often the term "sig" will appear just in front of these (short for the Latin, signetur, or "let it be labeled").

6. By what route (oral or otherwise) the medicine should be administered.

The mode of administration:

- **po** — from the Latin ***per os*****, or "by mouth" or "orally"**
- **pr** — from the Latin ***p**er **r**ectum,* or **"by way of the rectum,"** meaning by suppository
- **sl** — **s**ub**l**ingual (**under the tongue**)
- **IV** — **i**ntra**v**enously (**into a vein**)
- **IM** — **i**ntra**m**uscularly (**in the muscle**)
- **SC** — **s**ub**c**utaneously (**under the skin**)
- **ID**—**i**ntra**d**ermally (**between the layers of the skin**)

7. How often the medicine should be taken and other details about how to take it, such as time of day, or with or without food:

The frequency of administration:

- **qd** — **one/once a day**, from the Latin *quaque die*
- **bid** — **twice a day**, from the Latin *bis in die*
- **tid** — **three times a day**, from the Latin *ter in die*

- **qid — four times a day**, from the Latin *quater in die*
- **q4h — every 4 hours**, from the Latin *quaque 4 hora*
- **qh — every hour**, from the Latin *quaque hora*

If the medication is to be taken in a particular way — for example, at night, before food, or after food — that comes next

pc — after meals or **not on an empty stomach**, from the Latin *post cibum*

ac — before meals, from the Latin *ante cibum*

qhs — each night, from the Latin *quaque hora somni*, or **"at bedtime"**

prn — as needed, from the Latin *pro re nata*, "as circumstances may require"

For more information of prescription direction shorthand:

tab-tablet, from the Latin *tabella*

cap-capsule, from the Latin *capsula*

pil-pill, from the Latin *pilula*

syr-syrup

gtt-drop, from the Latin *gutta*

ung-ointment

cr-cream

od-right eye, from the Latin oculus *dexter*

os-left eye, from the Latin oculus *sinister*

tsp-teaspoon (5ml)

tbsp-tablespoon (15ml)

8. The number of doses to be dispensed at once (e.g., one month supply or more)

9. Number of refills:

The number of refills allowed is next. For example, it might say "3RF" for three refills.

10. DEA number:

For some prescriptions, but not all, additional information is required, including doctor's Drug Enforcement Agency (DEA) number. For example, certain controlled substances, including narcotics, require a valid DEA number.

11. Doctor's signature:

Words

the dosage of the medication: 약 성분 함량

identifying information: 개인 정보

at once/at one time: 한 번에

injections: 주사

and so on: 기타 등등

denote: 표기하다.

short for: ~의 약자로

Latin: 라틴어

let it be labeled: 표기하시오

after meals: 식 후

on an empty stomach: 공복에

before meals: 식 전

at bedtime/each night: 잠자리에 들 때

as needed/as circumstances may require: 필요 시

prescription direction: 처방전 복약지시

shorthand: 약자

drop: (안약과 같은) 점액

oral or otherwise: 경구 또는 다른 방법

the mode of administration: 투여 방법

per (=via, by): ~을 통하여

rectum: 직장

sublingual: 혀 아래의, 설하제(혀 아래에 약을 넣어 복용하는 법)

IV-intravenously: 정맥주사

IM-intramuscularly: 근육주사

SC-subcutaneouly: 피하주사

ID-intradermally: 피내주사

the frequency of administration: 복용빈도

one/once a day: 하루에 한 번

twice a day: 하루에 두 번

three times a day: 하루에 세 번

four times a day: 하루에 네 번

every 4 hours: 4시간 마다

dispensed at once: 한 번에 처방되는

one month supply: 한 달치 분량

refills: 의사에게서 처방전을 받지 않고 같은 약을 다시 조제 받는 것

Drug Enforcement Agency (DEA) number: 마약 단속반 번호

controlled substances: 규제 성분

narcotics: 마약성 진통제

valid: 유용한, 타당한

Drill: 아래의 빈칸에 알맞은 약자(Abbreviation)를 적어 넣으세요.

Abbreviation	Meaning	Latin Term
	before meals	ante cibum
	after meals	post cibum
	tablet	tabella
	capsule	capsula
	drop	gutta
	at bedtime	quaque hora somni
	right eye	oculus dexter
	left eye	oculus sinister
	by mouth	per os
	pill	pilula
	as needed	pro re nata
	every 2 hours	quaque 2 hora
	one/once a day	quaque die
	every hour	quaque hora
	4 times a day	quater in die
	twice a day	bis in die
	3 times a day	ter in die

Drill: How to read a prescription slip

처방전을 보고 아래의 질문(1-10)에 답하세요.

Mary Smith, M.D.
Family Practice
Small Town, USA

THIS DOCUMENT CONTAINS SECURITY BLACKPRINT

Name *John Doe* Age 53
①
Address *Small Town, USA* Date 01/19/04
②

③ ④
ibuprofen *600* mg

Sig: i *po* *qid* *pc* *prn*
⑤ ⑥ ⑦

\# *120* ⑧

Refill 3 times ⑨

⑩ DEA # 1234

⑪ *JohnDoe M.D.*

1. What are the patient's name, address, and date of birth/age?

Patient's name:____________________________________

Patient's address:__________________________________

Patient's date of birth/age:____________________________

2. What's the date today?

____

3. What's the name of the medication?

____

4. What's the dosage of the medication?

____

5. How many doses should the medicine be taken at once?

____

6. By what route (oral or otherwise) should the medicine be administered?

____

7. How often should the medicine be taken?

Also, are there any other details about how to take it, such as time of day, or with or without food?

____

If the medication is to be taken in a particular way — for example, at night, before food, or after food, then please describe it.

____

8. How many doses should the medicine be dispensed at once (e.g., one month supply or more)?

____

9. How many times can a patient get the prescription filled without getting his/her prescription issued again?

____

10. If the patient's prescription contains narcotic substances, please write down the DEA number.

____

Reading Material

Prescription Bottle

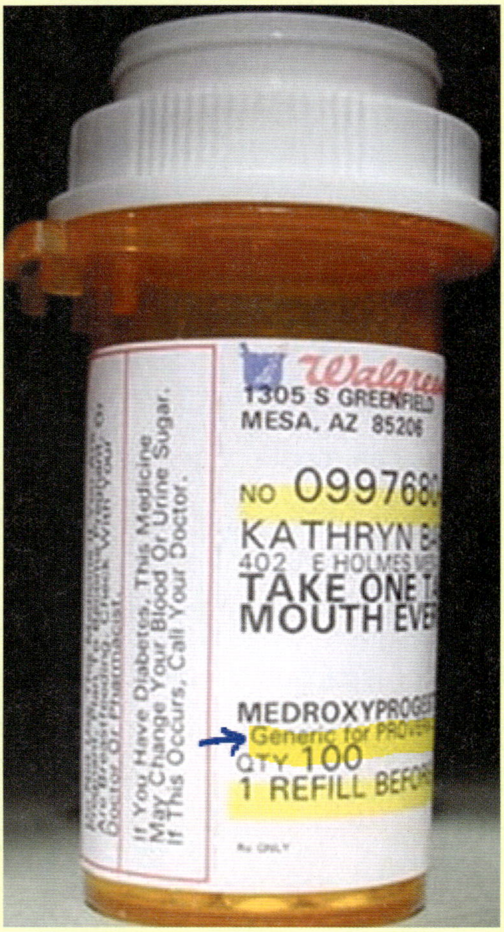

-->**Generic for Brand name drug**이란 환자가 오리지널약을 처방 받는 대신 카피약으로 처방을 의뢰함을 명시함.

What's on the prescription bottle label?

(Sample Prescription Bottle Label)

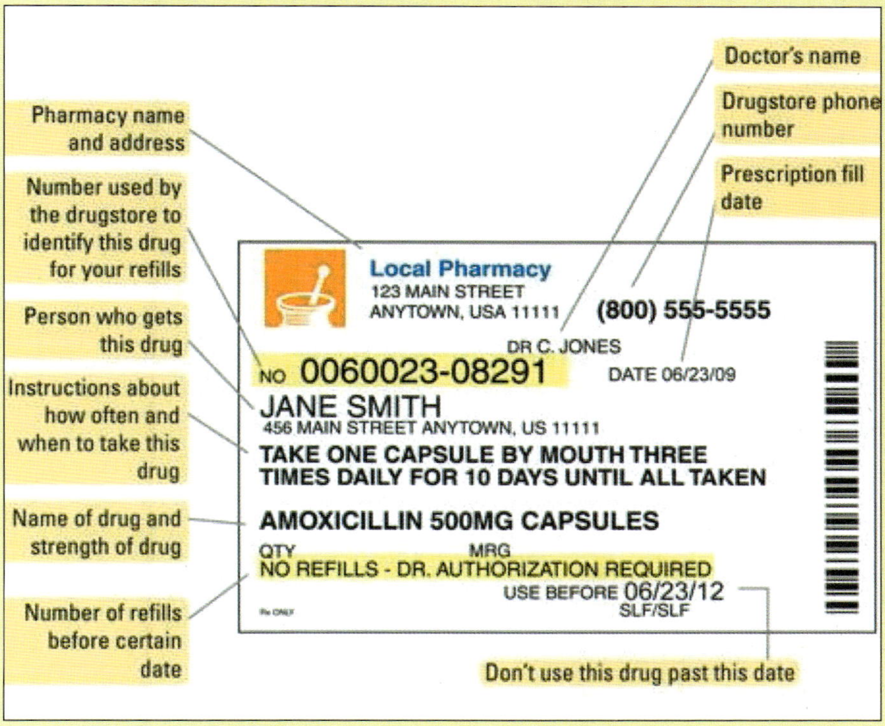

다음 페이지에 위의 Sample Prescription Bottle Label을 다시 적음

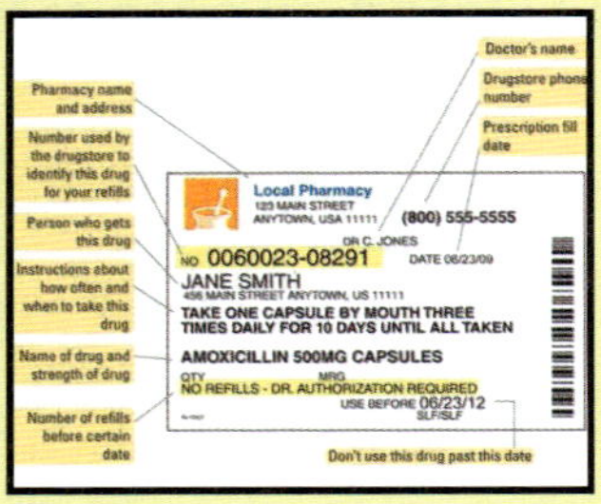

(Sample Prescription Bottle Label의 내용을 다시 적음)

Local Pharmacy
Pharmacy name and address

(800) 555-5555
Drugstore phone number

DR C. JONES
Doctor's name

NO 0060023-08291
Number used by the drug store to identify this drug for your refills

DATE 06/23/09
Prescription fill date

JANE SMITH
Person who gets this drug

TAKE ONE CAPSULE BY MOUTH THREE TIMES DAILY FOR 10 DAYS UNTIL ALL TAKEN
Instructions about how often and when to take this drug

AMOXICILLIN 500 MG CAPSULES
Name of drug and strength of drug

NO REFILLS
Number of refills before certain date

USE BEFORE 06/23/12
Don't use this drug past this date

Words

local: 그 지역의

refills: 재처방

strength of drug: 약의 함량

pharmacy/drugstore: 약국

NO 는 횟수를 의미함

past: 지난

Getting My Prescription Filled

At the doctor's office

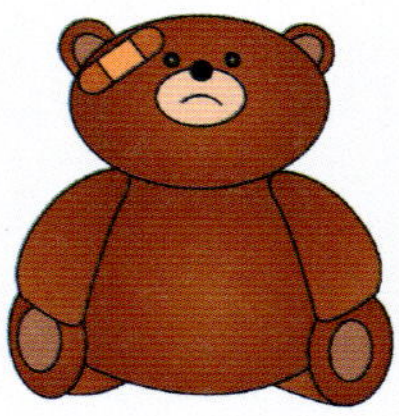

Dr. Mason: Mr. Smith, I am going to give you two prescriptions.
I've prescribed your medications for two weeks since you will go on a business trip to Korea for two weeks.

Mr. Smith: Thanks a lot. I really appreciate that.

Dr. Mason: Let me explain the medications that I prescribed to you. The first medication is an anti-inflammatory. This medication will reduce inflammation in your hip joints. You should take one tablet a day with a full glass of water as needed.

Mr. Smith: I see. Will it help to relieve my pain as well?

Dr. Mason: Yes.

Mr. Smith: Great.

Dr. Mason: The second medication is a water pill. Your blood pressure is still high, so I have prescribed a water pill to treat your hypertension. You should take one tablet once a day. Are you with me so far?

Mr. Smith: Yes, I am. Thank you.

Dr. Mason: You can pick up your prescription from the nurse on your way out. Do you have any other questions you'd like to ask?

Mr. Smith: No, I don't. Thanks a lot. I really appreciate it.

Dr. Mason: No problem. Have a nice trip.

Words

anti-inflammatory: 소염제

hip joints: 고관절

inflammation: 염증

water pill=diuretic: 이뇨제

hypertension=high blood pressure: 고혈압

Review: 각각의 구문을 영작하세요.
정답은 전 페이지의 Dialogue를 참고하세요.

Dr. Mason: 스미스 선생님, 두 가지 약을 처방해 드리겠습니다.

____

I've prescribed your medications for two weeks since you will go on a business trip to Korea for two weeks.
Mr. Smith: Thanks a lot. I really appreciate that.

Dr. Mason: 처방한 약에 관해 설명을 드리겠습니다.

____

첫 번째 약은 소염제입니다.

____

이 약은 고관절의 염증을 완화할 것입니다.

____

하루에 알약 한 알씩 충분한 양의 물과 필요할 때마다 복용하세요.

____

Mr. Smith: I see. Will it help to relieve my pain as well?

Dr. Mason: Yes.
Mr. Smith: Great.

Dr. Mason: 두 번째 약은 이뇨제입니다.

혈압이 아직도 높아요. 그래서 고혈압을 치료하기 위해 이뇨제를 처방했습니다.

하루에 한 알씩 복용하세요.

이해가 되셨습니까?

Mr. Smith: Yes, I am. Thank you.

Dr. Mason: 처방전은 밖에서 간호사 선생님한테 받아가세요.

다른 질문사항이 있나요?

Mr. Smith: No, I don't. Thanks a lot. I really appreciate it.

Dr. Mason: No problem. Have a nice trip.

3. Precautionary Measures on Taking Medication 복약지시에 관한 주의사항

- **Key Expressions for Precautionary Measures on Taking Medication, 복약지시에 관한 주의사항 관련 주요구문**

  - Words, 어휘
  - Drill, 연습문제

Key Expressions for Precautionary Measures on Taking Medication

Please don't ~

1. **Please don't drink alcoholic beverages or smoke** while taking this medication.

2. **Please do not take this medication with other medicines.**

3. **Please don't forget to take** your medicines.

4. **Please avoid dairy products** while taking your antibiotics (Diet exclusion).

5. **Do not consume your medicines** on an empty stomach.

6. **Please complete the full course of** prescribed medicines.

7. **Please do not leave** once you start feeling better. Incomplete treatment might welcome the disease again.

8. **Please take your medications** at the same time every day if it's possible.

9. **Please don't lie down** for 30 minutes after taking your osteoporosis medication. For this reason, **please don't take** it right before bedtime.

10. **Please take your medication** with food to lessen stomach upset.

Words

alcoholic beverages: 술, 알코올을 포함한 모든 음료

dairy products: 유제품

diet exclusion: 제한해야 할 음식

on an empty stomach: 공복에

the full course of: 전부

osteoporosis medication: 골다공증 약

lessen: ~을 완화시키다.

Drill: Q1-Q11은 Fill in the blanks 문제입니다. 알맞은 구문을 넣어 완성하세요.

정답은 전 페이지의 Key Expressions을 참고하세요.

Fill in the blanks

Q1. ____ while taking this medication.

이 약을 복용하시는 동안에 술 또는 담배를 피하세요.

Q2. Please do not take this medication ________________.

이 약을 다른 약과 함께 복용하지 마세요.

Q3. _____________________________take your medicines.

잊지 말고 약을 복용하세요.

Q4. _______________________________ while taking your antibiotics.

항생제를 복용할 때 유제품을 피하세요.

Q5. Do not consume your medicines_____________________.

공복에 약을 복용하지 마세요.

Q6. ________________________________prescribed

medicines.

처방 받은 약을 끝까지 다 복용하세요

Q7. Please do not leave__________________________.

차도가 있다고 복약을 중단하지 마세요.

Q8. Please take your ___________________________

__________________________if it's possible.

가급적이면 매일 같은 시간에 약을 복용하세요.

Q9. ____

osteoporosis medication.

골다공증 약을 복용한 후 30분 동안은 눕지 마세요.

Q10. Please don't take it__________________________.

잠자리에 들기 바로 전에 이 약을 복용하지 마세요.

Q11. Please take your medication ___________________.

속 쓰림을 줄이기 위해 음식과 함께 복용하세요.

4. How to Take My Medications
약을 복용하는 방법

- **A List of Key Expressions, 주요구문 모음**

A. How often should I take it?/How many pills should I take?: 얼마나 자주 복용해야 하나요?/몇 알씩 복용해야 하나요?

- Words, 어휘
- Drill, 연습문제

B. 30 Minutes before meals, 식사 전 30분 복용

- Dialogue, 대화
- Words, 어휘
- Drill, 연습문제

C. 30 Minutes after meals, 식사 후 30분 복용

- Dialogue, 대화
- Words, 어휘
- Drill, 연습문제

D. With your meals/Right after meals: 식사와 함께/식사 후 즉시 복용

- Dialogue, 대화
- Drill, 연습문제

E. Before Going to Bed: 취침 전에 복용

- Dialogue, 대화
- Words, 어휘
- Drill, 연습문제

F. As Needed: 필요할 때마다 복용

- Dialogue, 대화
- Words, 어휘
- Drill, 연습문제

- **Reading Material: The right way to take an antibiotic, 독해구문: 항생제의 올바른 복용방법**

    - Words, 어휘
    - Drill, 연습문제

A List of Key Expressions

A. How often should I take it? How many pills should I take?

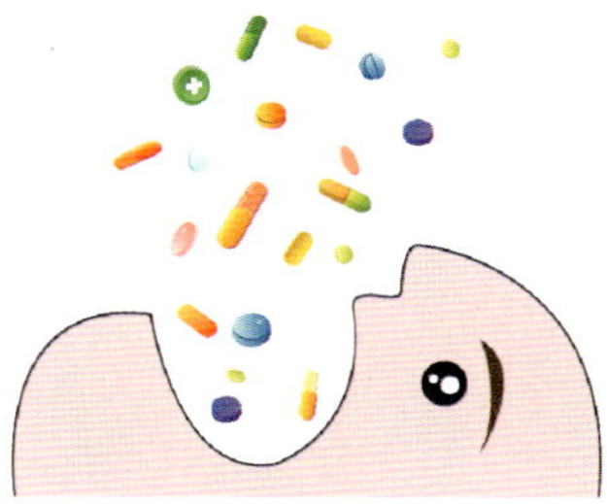

1. You need to take one pill **three times a day.**

2. You need to take the medication **every other day.**

3. You need to take your hair growth pill **every five days.**

4. You take two of these capsules **after every meal three times a day.**

5. My prescription says to take my pain medication **every 4 hours.**

6. You need to take Fosamax Plus tablet **with a full glass of water once a week.**

7. Please take your medicine **as needed.**

Words

every other day: 2틀에 한 번

hair growth pill: 발모제

every meal: 식사할 때마다

my prescription says: 처방전에 따르면

a full glass of water: 충분한 양의 물

as needed: 필요할 때마다

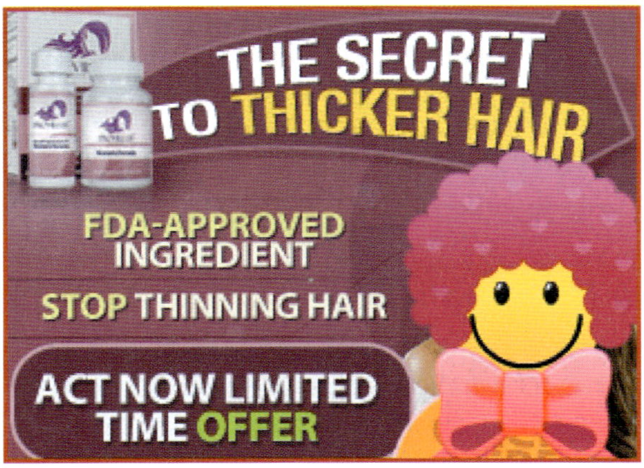
THE SECRET
TO THICKER HAIR
FDA-APPROVED
INGREDIENT
STOP THINNING HAIR
ACT NOW LIMITED
TIME OFFER

TIP

Thicker Hair: 머리 숱이 많은

Stop Thinning Hair: 머리 숱이 적어지는 것을 방지

FDA-Approved Ingredient: 미 식약청이 승인한 약 성분을 사용

Drill: Q1-Q7을 영작하세요

정답은 A List of Key Expressions를 페이지를 참고하세요.

Q1. 알약 한 알을 하루에 세 번씩 복용하세요.

____

Q2. 이 약을 2틀에 한 번씩 복용하세요.

____

Q3. 발모제를 5일에 한 번씩 복용하세요.

____

Q4. 매번 식사 후 캡슐 두 알을 하루에 세 번씩 복용하세요.

____

Q5. 처방전에 따르면 네 시간마다 진통제를 복용하라고 적혀 있습니다.

____

Q6. 포사맥스 플러스정(골다공증 치료약)을 일주일에 한 번 충분한 양의 물과 함께 복용하세요.

____

Q7. 필요할 때마다 복용하세요.

____

A List of Key Expressions

B. 30 minutes before meals

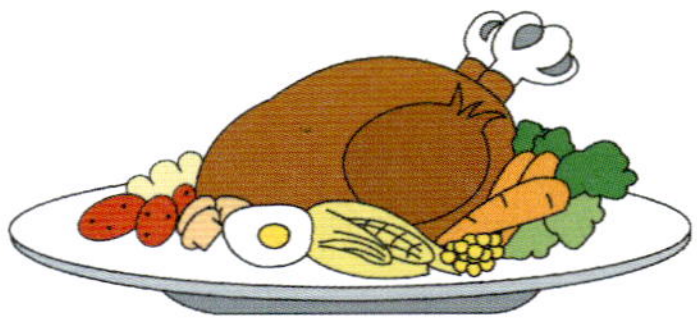

1. Please take your medicine **approximately 30 minutes before your meals.**

2. Please take two tablets **half an hour before the meals.**

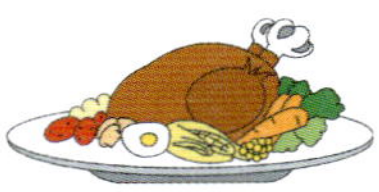

Jason: How often should you take your meds?

Jane: My pharmacist told me to take two pills half an hour before each meal.

Words

half an hour: 30분

meds=medications/medicines: 약을 가볍게 표현한 다른 말

Drill: Q1-Q4를 영작하세요

정답은 A List of Key Expressions를 참고하세요.

Q1. 식사하기 약 30분 전에 약을 복용하세요.

____

Q2. 식사하기 30분 전에 알약을 두 개씩 복용하세요.

____

Q3. 당신은 얼마나 자주 약을 복용해야 하나요?

____

Q4. 약사 선생님이 식사하기 30분 전에 알약을 두 개씩 복용하라고 했어요.

____

A List of Key Expressions

C. 30 minutes after meals

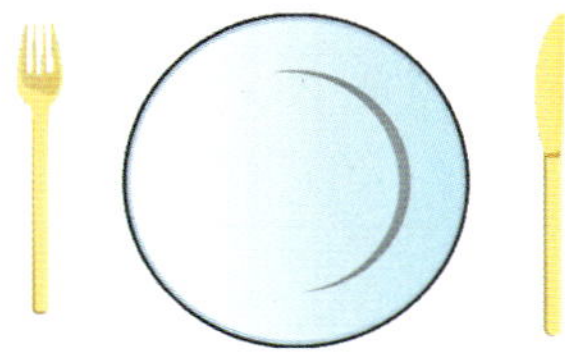

1. Please take three tablets with a full glass of water **30 minutes after meals.**

2. Please take two tablespoons of cough syrup three times a day **half an hour after each meal.**

Patient: When is the best time for me to take my antibiotic medications?

Pharmacist: Well, the best time to take your antibiotic medication is 30 minutes after every meal. There is a list of precautionary measures on your prescription bottle. It says that you don't take your antibiotics on an empty stomach because it can irritate the lining of your stomach, so please take it about 30 minutes after your meals.

Words

antibiotic medications: 항생제

precautionary measures: 주의사항

on an empty stomach: 공복에

irritate: 속을 쓰리게 하다

the lining of your stomach: 위벽

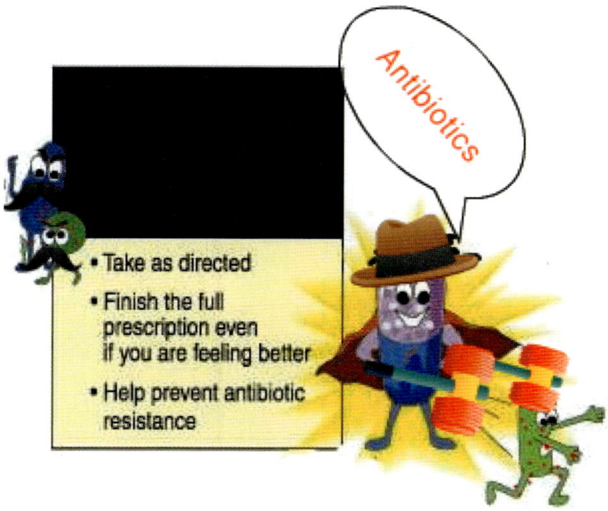

Take as directed: 복약지시에 따라 복용하시오.

Finish the full prescription even if you are feeling better: 차도가 있을지라도 처방 받은 항생제를 모두 복용하시오.

Help prevent antibiotic resistance: 항생제에 내성이 생기지 않도록 하시오.

Drill: Q1-Q6을 영작하세요

정답은 A List of Key Expressions를 참고하세요.

Q1. 식사하고 30분 후에 알약 세 개를 충분한 양의 물과 함께 복용하세요.

____

Q2. 식후 30분 뒤에 기침시럽 두 스푼을 하루에 세 번 복용하세요.

____

Q3. 항생제를 복용하기에 가장 좋은 시간이 언제인가요?

____

Q4. 항생제 복용에 가장 좋은 시간은 매 식사 후 30분 뒤입니다.

____

Q5. 약병에 주의사항들이 적혀 있습니다.

____

Q6. 위벽을 상하게 할 수 있으니 항생제를 공복에 복용하지 말도록 여기 적혀 있으므로, 식후 30분 뒤에 복용하세요.

____

____

A List of Key Expressions

D. With your meals/Right after meals

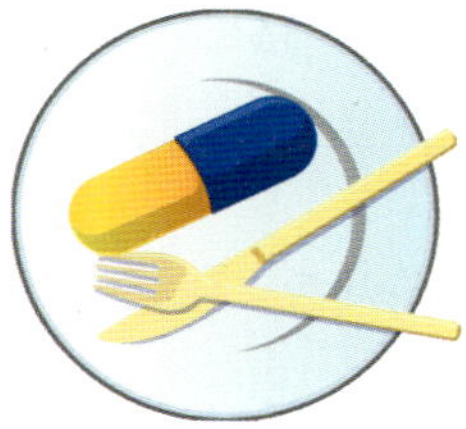

1. Please take this medication **right after each meal.**

2. Please take your medication **at the same time as you have your meal.**

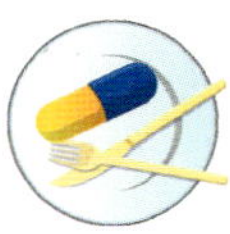

Max: Dinner is ready. Linda, would you please bring my medication for me?

Linda: Sure. By the way, are you taking your medication with your meal?

Max: Yes, I am. My doctor told me to take my pills with food, so I should take them at the same time as I have my meal every day.

Drill: Q1-Q4를 영작하세요

정답은 A List of Key Expressions를 참고하세요.

Q1. 이 약을 식 후 바로 복용하세요.

____

Q2. 약을 식사와 함께 복용하세요.

____

Q3. 그런데 당신은 약을 식사와 함께 복용하나요?

____

Q4. 의사선생님이 음식과 함께 복용하라고 해서, 매일 식사시간에 복용해야 해요.

____

A List of Key Expressions

E. Before going to bed

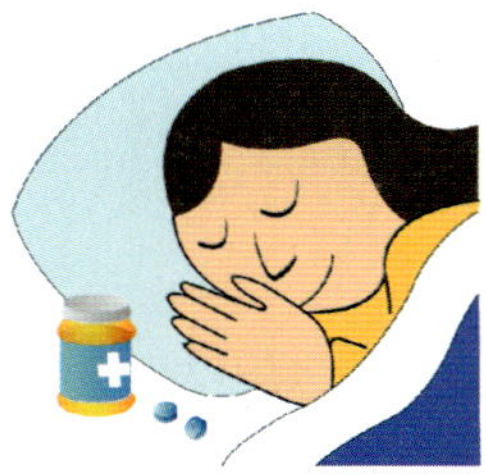

1. Please take your sleeping pill **about 30 minutes before you go to bed.**

2. Please take your night time medication **half an hour before going to bed.**

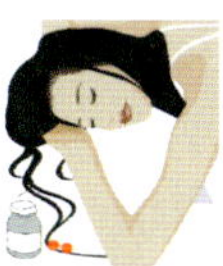

Herb doctor: How can I help you?

Patient: Well, I couldn't sleep through the night for about a month, but I don't want to take any prescription sleeping pills or over-the-counter sleeping aids. I am kind of worried about the fact that they carry the side effects and can be habit-forming. Can you recommend me better sleeping pills, doctor?

Chapter 6

Herb doctor: Well, I recommend you a natural sleep aid. Natural sleep aids do not usually have side effects, and they are non-habit forming. Would you like to try them?

Patient: Yes. I will give it a shot.

Words

over-the-counter sleeping aids: 비 처방전 수면제

habit-forming: 습관성

a natural sleep aid: 내추럴(생약성분) 수면제

give it a shot(give it a go): ~을 해보겠다.

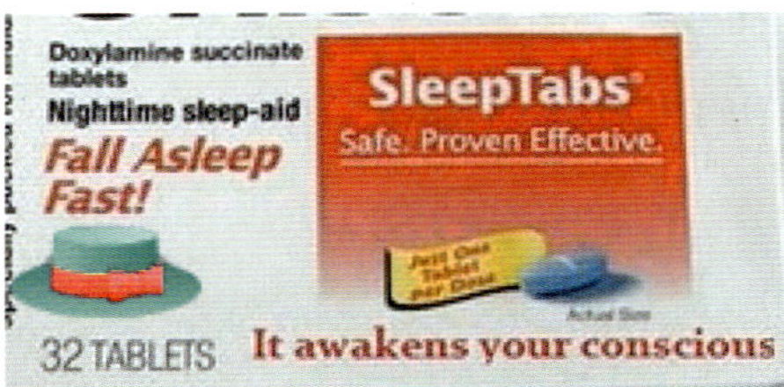

TIP

Proven Effective: 효과가 입증된

Night time Sleep-aid: 수면제

Fall Asleep Fast: 빨리 잠이 드는

Drill: Q1-Q7을 영작하세요

정답은 A List of Key Expressions를 참고하세요.

Q1. 잠자기 30분 전에 수면제를 복용하세요.

____

Q2. 밤에 복용하는 약은 잠자기 30분 전에 드세요.

____

Q3. 수면제를 처방 받거나, 처방전 없이 구할 수 있는 수면제를 복용하고 싶지 않습니다.

____

Q4. 수면제가 부작용이 있고 습관성이 될 수 있다는 사실이 염려됩니다.

____

Q5. 더 나은 수면제를 추천해 주실 수 있습니까?

____

Q6. 그러면 내츄럴(생약성분) 수면제를 추천해 드리겠습니다.

____

Q7. 내츄럴(생약성분) 수면제는 거의 부작용이 없고 습관성이 되지 않습니다.

____

A List of Key Expressions

F. As needed

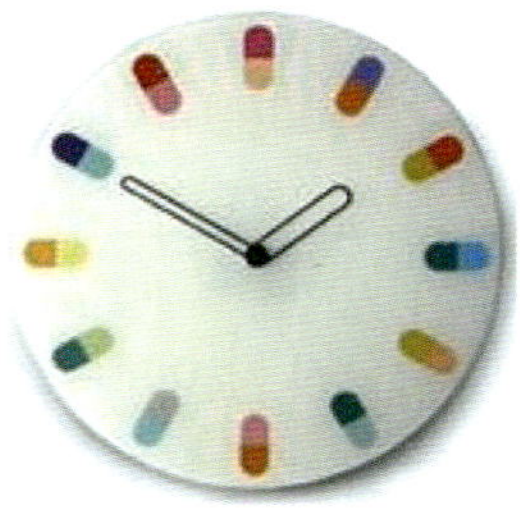

1. Please take your medicine **as needed to relieve your symptoms as they arise.**

2. You need to take your medication every 6 to 8 hours **as needed for pain.**

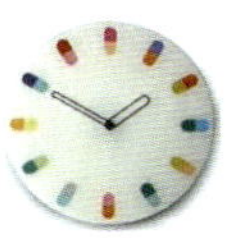

Patient: I am suffering from dry cough and a sore throat for about a week. Can you recommend me a good lozenge or throat spray?

Pharmacist: Sure. I recommend this lozenge. It will soothe your sore throat and suppress your dry cough. Please take your throat lozenge as needed to relieve your symptoms as they arise. However, if your cough goes on and on and gets worse instead of getting better, make sure you see a doctor.

Patient: I see. Thank you.

Pharmacist: No problem.

Words

dry cough: 마른기침

sore throat: 인후염

lozenge: 목 캔디

throat spray: 목에 뿌리는 감기약

suppress: 억제하다

soothe: ~을 진정시키다.

goes on and on: 계속 지속되고

Anti-Snore Spray

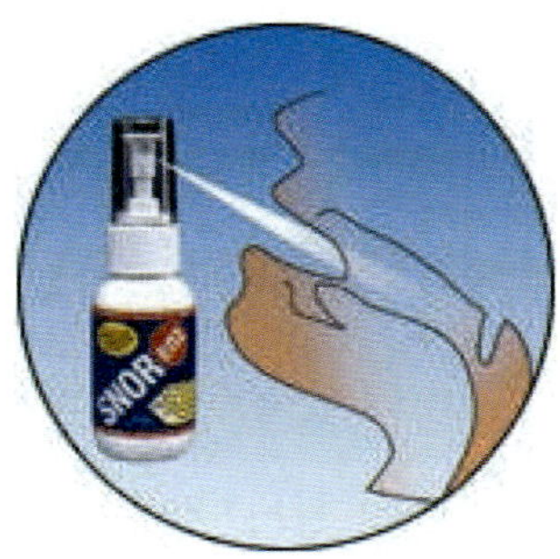

Fast Effective Relief

Stop Snoring Now!

TIP

Throat Spray: 목에 뿌리는 감기약

Anti-Snore Spray: 코고는 것을 방지하기 위해 뿌리는 약

Fast Effective Relief: 효과가 빠른

Stop Snoring Now: 코 고는 것을 당장 멈춤

Drill: Q1-Q7를 영작하세요

정답은 A List of Key Expressions를 참고하세요.

Q1. 증상을 완화시키기 위해 필요할 때마다 약을 복용하세요.

____

Q2. 통증을 완화시키기 위해 6-8시간 간격으로 필요할 때마다 약을 복용하세요.

____

Q3. 약 일주일 동안 마른기침과 인후염으로 고생하고 있습니다.

____

Q4. 잘 듣는 목 캔디나 목 스프레이를 추천해 주시겠습니까?

____

Q5. 이것은 인후염을 진정시키고, 마른 기침을 제거해줄 것입니다.

____

Q6. 증상을 완화하기 위해 필요할 때마다 이 목 캔디를 드세요.

____

Q7. 하지만, 기침이 계속 지속되고 차도가 있는 대신 더 악화되면 진료를 받으세요.

____

Reading Material

The right way to take an antibiotic

You have filled a prescription for an antibiotic. If you use an antibiotic the wrong way, it can make infection stronger and harder to treat. Please read the following important information.

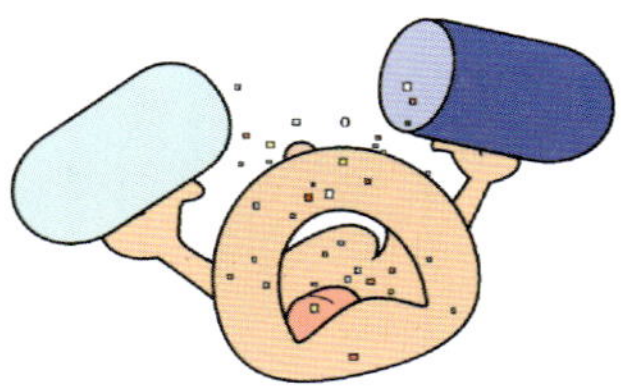

- **Please take your antibiotics the right way**
- **Please take it as your medical provider tells you**
- **Please do not skip doses**
- **Please do not share it with others**
- **Please do not save it for later**
- **Please finish your prescription even if you feel better**

Words

filled a prescription: 약을 처방 받다.

antibiotic: 항생제

wrong way: 잘못된 방법

infection: 감염

medical provider: 의료진

skip doses: 복용을 거르다.

save: 남겨두다

feel better: 차도가 있다.

Drill: Q1-Q6을 영작하세요.

정답은 The right way to take an antibiotic을 참고하세요.

Q1. 항생제를 올바른 방법으로 복용하세요.

____

Q2. 의료진들이 설명한대로 항생제를 복용하세요.

____

Q3. 항생제 복용하는 것을 거르지 마세요.

____

Q4. 다른 사람과 함께 복용하지 마세요.

____

Q5. 나중에 사용하기 위해 남겨놓지 마세요.

____

Q6. 상태가 호전되더라도 처방 받은 항생제를 다 드세요.

____

5. FAQ at the Pharmacy 약국에서 자주하는 질문

- **A List of FAQ at the pharmacy, 약국에서 자주하는 질문 모음**
    - Words, 어휘
    - Drill, 연습문제

A List of FAQ at the Pharmacy

Patient: Are there any precautionary measures before I take the medicine?

Pharmacist: Yes. Please do not take this medicine on an empty stomach.

Patient: Should I stop drinking alcoholic beverages while I am taking this medication?

Pharmacist: Yes. You are not allowed to drink any alcohol while you are on this medication.

Patient: Can you tell me the administration schedule?

Pharmacist: It's on the prescription bottle, so please take your medication as directed.

Patient: **How can I remember to take my medicine?**

Pharmacist: You can use special pill boxes which are like the day-of-the-week divided ones found at drugstores. That will help you keep track.

Patient: **How should I apply this ointment?**

Pharmacist: Apply a thin coat of this ointment every morning and then cover it with a dressing.

Patient: **Should I store my medications in the refrigerator to keep them cool?**

Pharmacist: Please store your medication at room temperature and away from excess heat and moisture (not in the bathroom). Also, you should keep your medication in the container it came in, tightly closed, and out of the reach of children. You need to store your medicine the way your doctor or pharmacist tells you.

Patient: **Can I stop taking these medicines if I feel better?**

Pharmacist: Don't stop taking them suddenly without the approval of your doctor. Please keep taking them regularly until all is gone.

Patient: Do you think I can drive a car after taking this medication?

Pharmacist: It is best not to drive a car, because you may feel sleepy or drowsy after you take this medicine.

Patient: How do I get my prescription filled?

Pharmacist: Simply bring your prescription to a pharmacy and have it filled.

Patient: Do you carry throat logenzies and merthiolate?

Pharmacist: Yes, we do.

Words

precautionary measures: 주의사항, 예방책

on an empty stomach: 공복에

alcoholic beverages: 알코올성 음료, 술

on this medication: 약을 복용 중에

the day-of-the-week divided: 일주일이 각각 나뉘어진

keep track: 기억할 수 있는

apply: 연고를 바르다

apply a thin coat: 얇게 펴 바르세요

store: ~을 보관하다

at room temperature: 실내온도

feel better: 차도가 있다

sleepy or drowsy: 졸린

get one's prescription filled: ~의 약을 처방전대로 받다

have it filled: 약을 처방 받다

carry: (가게에서) ~을 판매하다

merthiolate: (외상에 바르는 빨간색) 소독약

Drill: Q1-Q11은 Fill in the blanks 문제입니다. 알맞은 구문을 넣어 완성하세요. Q12-Q22의 FAQ를 영작하세요.
정답은 전 페이지의 A List of FAQ at the Pharmacy를 참고하세요.

Fill in the blanks

Q1. Are there any ____________________ before I take the medicine?

제가 이 약을 복용하기 전에 주의해야 할 사항이 있나요?

Q2. Please do not take this medicine____________________.

이 약을 공복에 복용하지 마세요.

Q3. Should I stop drinking alcoholic beverages ____________________?

이 약을 복용 중에 금주해야 하나요?

Q4. Can you tell me ____________________?

약 복용법을 알려주시겠습니까?

Q5. How can I remember ____________________?

약 복용하는 것을 어떻게 기억할 수 있을까요?

Q6. How should I ______________________________?

이 연고를 어떻게 바르나요?

Q7. ______________________ in the refrigerator to keep them cool?

제 약을 냉장고에 보관해야 하나요?

Q8. Can I stop taking these medicines ________________?

만일 차도가 있으면 복용을 중단해도 되나요?

Q9. Do you think I can drive a car ________________?

이 약을 복용한 후 운전을 해도 되나요?

Q10. How do I ______________________________?

약을 어떻게 처방 받지요?

Q11. Do you carry ____________________________?

목 캔디와 소독약 팔아요?

FAQ

Q12. 이 약을 공복에 복용하지 마세요.

____

Q13. 처방 받은 약병에 적혀 있습니다. 복약지시대로 드시면 됩니다.

Q14. 일주일 분량의 약을 요일 별로 나누어 담는 용기를 약국에서 구입하세요.

Q15. 매일 아침 얇게 연고를 바르시고 거즈를 붙이세요.

Q16. 실내온도로 보관하시고 지나친 열기 및 습기가 있는 곳은 피하세요(화장실에 보관하지 마세요).

Q17. 또한 약은 원래의 약병에 밀폐시켜서 보관하시고, 어린이들의 손에 닿지 않는 곳에 보관 하세요.

Q18. 약은 의사 또는 약사의 지시에 따라 보관하세요.

Q19. 의사선생님의 승인 없이는 갑자기 중단하지 마세요.

Q20. 다 드실 때까지 규칙적으로 복용하세요.

____

Q21. 이 약을 복용한 후 졸릴 수 있으므로 운전은 하지 않는 것이 최선입니다.

____

Q22. 처방전을 약국에 가져오시고 약을 받으시면 됩니다.

____

6. Over-the-Counter Medication
비처방전 약

- **Reading Material, 독해구문**
  - Over-The-Counter Medication Label, 비처방전 약 설명서
  - What does OTC label say?, 비처방전 약 설명서에는 무엇이 기재되어 있나요?
  - Words, 어휘
- **Getting My OTC Medication, 비처방전 약 구매**
  - Dialogue, 대화
  - Words, 어휘
  - Review, 복습

Reading Material

Over-The-Counter Medicaton Label

Drug Facts

Active ingredient (in each tablet)	***Purpose***
Chlorpheniramine maleate 2 mg	Antihistamine

Uses temporarily relieves these symptoms due to hay fever or other upper respiratory allerigies:
- sneezing
- runny nose
- itchy, watery eyes
- itchy throat

Warnings

Ask a doctor before use if you have
- glaucoma
- a breathing problem such as emphysema or chronic bronchitis
- trouble urinating due to an enlarged prostate gland

Ask a doctor or pharmacist before use if you are taking tranquilizers or sedatives

When using this procuct
- You may get drowsy
- Avoid alcoholic drinks
- Alcohol, sedatives, and tranquilizers may increase drowsiness
- Be careful when driving a motor vehicle or operating machinery
- Excitability may occur, especially in children

If pregnant or breastfeeding, ask a health professional before use.

Keep out of reach of children. In case of overdose, get medical help or contact a Poison Control Center right away.

Directions

Adults and children 12 years and over	Take 2 tablets every 4 to 6 hours; not more than 12 tablets in 24 hours
Children 6 years to under 12 years	Take 1 tablet every 4 to 6 hours; not more than 6 tablets in 24 hours
Children under 6 years	Ask a doctor

Other information Store at 20-25° C (68-77° F)
- Protect from excessive moisture

Inactive ingredients D&C yellow no. 10, lactose, magnesium stearate, microcrystalline cellulose, pregelatinized starch

다음 페이지에 위의 Sample Prescription Bottle Label 을 다시 적음

What does OTC label say?

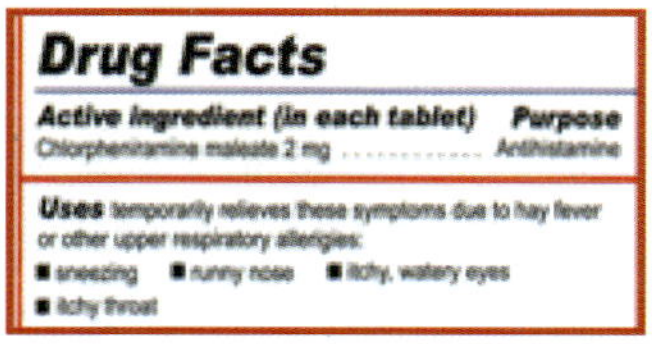

Drug Facts
Active ingredient (in each tablet) Purpose
Chlorpheniramine maleate 2 mg .... Antihistamine
Uses temporarily relieves these symptoms due to hay fever or other upper respiratory allergies:
■ sneezing ■ runny nose ■ itchy, watery eyes
■ itchy throat

(OTC Medication Label Sample을 다시 적음)

Drug Facts:

Active ingredient (in each tablet) **Purpose**

Chlorpheniramine maleate 2 mg ....Antihistamine

---

Uses temporarily relieves these symptoms due to hay fever or other upper respiratory allergies:

- sneezing
- runny nose
- itchy, watery eyes
- itchy throat

Warnings

Ask a doctor before use if you have

- glaucoma
- a breathing problem such as emphysema or chronic bronchitis
- trouble urinating due to an enlarged prostate gland

Ask a doctor or pharmacist before use if you are taking tranquilizers or sedatives

When using this product

- You may get drowsy
- Avoid alcoholic drinks
- Alcohol, sedatives, and tranquilizers may increase drowsiness
- Be careful when driving a motor vehicle or operating machinery
- Excitability may occur, especially in children

If pregnant or breastfeeding, ask a health professional before use.

Keep out of reach of children. In case of overdose, get medical help or contact a Poison Control Center right away.

Directions

Adults and children 12 years and over	Take 2 tablets every 4 to 6 hours; not more than 12 tablets in 24 hours
Children 6 years to under 12 years	Take 1 tablet every 4 to 6 hours; not more than 6 tablets in 24 hours
Children under 6 years	Ask a doctor

Other information store at 20-25°C (68-77°F)

- protect from excessive moisture

Inactive ingredients

D&C yellow no. 10, lactose, magnesium stearate, microcrystalline cellulose, pregelatinized starch

Source: http://www.womenshealth.gov

Words

Drug Facts: 약의 정보

temporarily relieves: 일시적으로 증상을 완화시킨다.

hay fever: 꽃가루 앨러지

upper respiratory allergies: 상기도 호흡기 앨러지

itchy throat: 간질거리는 목

glaucoma: 녹내장

emphysema: 기관지 확장증

chronic bronchitis: 만성기관지염

urinating: 배뇨

prostate gland: 전립선

tranquilizers: 신경안정제

sedatives: 진정제

excitability: 흥분 상태

breastfeeding: 모유 수유

overdose: 과다 복용

every 4 to 6 hours: 4시간에서 6시간 마다

store: 보관하세요

excessive moisture: 지나치게 습기가 많은 곳

pregelatinized starch: 호화(알파)전분

Getting My OTC Medication

OTC Decongestant

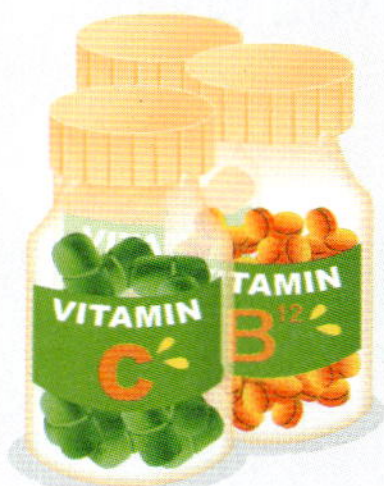

Pharmacist: How may I help you?

Customer: I've had a stuffy nose for a couple of days. Can you recommend a good nasal decongestant?

Pharmacist: I recommend this decongestant. It is very effective.

Customer: Great. How many tablets do I need to take?

Pharmacist: You need to take three tablets for each day.

Customer: Um. I am very forgetful, so I am worried what if I miss a dose?

Pharmacist: Well, if you miss a dose, please take it as soon as remembered if it is within an hour.

Customer: I see. However, if I do not remember until later, then do I need to double-up my doses to make up for the missed one?

Pharmacist: You should skip the missed dose and resume your usual dosing schedule, but you will not double-up the doses. Do you understand?
Customer: Yes, I do. By the way, are there any side effects?

Pharmacist: Well, some patients have reported slight dizziness and queasy feeling. Also, it causes drowsiness, so you shouldn't drive a car after taking this medication.
Customer: I won't.

Pharmacist: Do you have any other questions?
Customer: No. Thanks a lot. I really appreciate it.

Pharmacist: No problem. But if it gets any worse, then you should see your doctor.

Words

stuffy nose: 코가 막힘

decongestant: 코 막힘을 풀어주는 약

I am very forgetful: 나는 건망증이 심해요.

within an hour: 한 시간 이내

make up: 보충하다.

double-up the doses: 복용량을 두 배로

queasy feeling: 메스꺼움, 오심

gets any worse: 더 악화된다면

Review: 각각의 구문을 영작하세요.

정답은 전 페이지의 Dialogue를 참고하세요.

Pharmacist: How may I help you?

Customer: I've had a stuffy nose for a couple of days.

코 막힌데 좋은 약을 추천해 주시겠습니까?

____

Pharmacist: 이 코막힘 약을 추천해 드리겠습니다.

____

매우 효과적입니다.

____

Customer: Great. How many tablets do I need to take?

Pharmacist: 하루에 세 알씩 드세요.

____

Customer: 음. 제가 건망증이 심해요. 그래서 만일에 약 복용하는 것을 잊으면 어떻게 하나요?

____

Pharmacist: 음. 만일 복용량을 한번 걸렀고, 한 시간 안에 기억한다면, 곧바로 드세요.

____

Customer: 알겠습니다. 하지만 한참 후에 기억한다면, 복용을 하지 못한 약을 함께 두 배로 복용해야 하나요?

Pharmacist: 복용하지 못한 약은 거르시고 다시 복용 일정을 따라주세요. 그리고 결코 약을 두 배로 복용하지 마세요.

Do you understand?

Customer: 예 그런데 부작용이 있나요?

Pharmacist: 음, 일부 환자들이 어지러움과 메스꺼움을 호소했습니다.

또한, 이 약은 졸음을 유발하므로, 복용 후 운전하지 마세요.

Customer: I won't.

Pharmacist: Do you have any other questions?

Customer: No. Thanks a lot. I really appreciate it.

Pharmacist: No problem. But if it gets any worse, then you should see your doctor.

7. 정답 및 해석

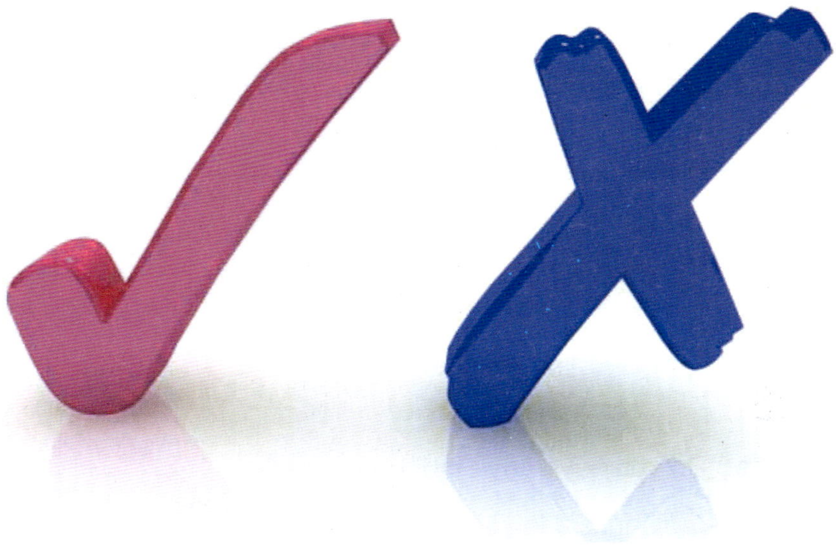

1. 주요어휘

약국과 관련된 연습문제 정답

M	C	G	X	O	I	A	E	K	S	O	T	D	E	G	X	M
T	M	E	T	D	R	L	P	X	X	N	Q	T	Y	U	B	U
P	B	N	W	Q	L	L	V	L	N	B	F	Q	C	R	L	E
T	H	E	R	A	P	E	U	T	I	C	K	C	A	M	Y	S
X	P	R	E	S	C	R	I	P	T	I	O	N	J	E	G	O
G	X	I	H	D	F	G	S	A	D	H	D	U	D	I	X	Y
S	M	C	Y	K	L	I	N	B	N		N	R	K	H	Q	N
U	D		O	N	L	C	M	Q	N	T	O	I	E	J	X	Q
J	B	D	H	E	R		F	A	O	P	R	C	I	U	U	J
E	E	R	B	R	Y	R	M	U	P	O	E	P	Q	Y	B	G
E	S	U	S	I	D	E		E	F	F	E	C	T	S	G	H
A	U	G	F	P		A	R	O	N	L	J	Q	R	D	O	Y
D	G	M	E	D	I	C	A	T	I	O	N		V	I	A	L
J	D	I	R	N	W	T	Y	E	J	N	G	L	K	H	Q	T
S	J	U	B	K	U	I	S	O	V	O	K	H	O	C	C	F
A	G	L	F	P	O	O	V	E	R	D	O	S	E	G	A	V
M	G	G	R	A	I	N		S	P	O	O	N	D	B	C	M

Prescription	Generic drug	Brand name drug
Allergic reaction	Therapeutic	Medication vial
grain spoon	Overdose	Eyedropper
Side effects		

1. 주요어휘
약의 종류와 관련된 연습문제 정답

X	X	S	N	Y	S	O	I	N	T	M	E	N	T	L	G	I	W
K	W	Q	A	P	M	N	N	Q	R	U	E	B	M	S	M	L	B
I	K	Q	T	F	G	O	M	A	A	V	O	J	J	B	I	C	A
W	A	C	U	T	H	C	F	W	N	X	K	C	Y	Q	J	W	S
J	B	U	R	L	R	D	E	C	S	R	T	C	U	H	L	M	Q
X	B	J	A	F	M	S	J	Y	D	M	S	I	K	X	L	M	L
D	P	X	L	V	M	U	O	B	E	V	D	P	B	F	C	F	I
L	V	P		J	L	P	H	B	R		V	L	S	J	X	H	T
E	X	B	M	R	D	P	V	N	M	M	D	A	A	E	B	F	Y
E	I	Q	E	A	M	O	H	E	A	E	R	R	W	K	M	V	U
P	U	O	D	L	L	S	D	E	L	K	X	I	O	A	U	I	C
I	M	I	I	P	J	I	X	L		N	M	G	S	P	X	X	H
T	C	I	C	H	C	T	B	D	P	N	X	O	H	B	S	Y	F
K	K	F	A	A	Y	O	J	C	A	C	L	M	N	N	E	I	N
E	D	Q	T	X	K	R	T	G	T	Q	N	G	D	U	P	M	P
E	B	I	I	B	A	Y	P	Y	C	A	O	L	C	U	U	X	K
N	O	L	O	Z	E	N	G	E	H	U	X	G	W	I	O	F	P
N	M	A	N	T	I	T	U	S	S	I	V	E	S	U	L	N	F

Suppository
Antitussives
Ointment
Liquid medication
Natural medication
Eye drops
Lozenge
Transdermal patch

1. 주요어휘
약 이름에 관한 연습문제 정답

1. (Diuretic/Water pill, 이뇨제)

2. (Throat lozenge, 목 캔디)

3. (Hemorrhoid relief cream, 치질연고)

4. (Back patch, 등에 부치는 파스)

5. (Sleeping aid/Sleeping pill, 수면제)

6. (Antacid, 제산제)

7. (Lubricant eye drops/Dry eye relief/Artificial tears: 인공눈물)

8. (Motion sickness relief medication: 멀미약)

1. 주요어휘
대화

약국에서

Pharmacist: 좋은 아침입니다. 무엇을 도와 드릴까요?
Mr. Smith: 예. 처방전대로 약을 지어주세요.

Pharmacist: 알겠습니다. 처방전을 보여 주세요.
Mr. Smith: 네, 여기 있습니다. 음, 그리고 치실과 챕스틱도 필요합니다. 어디에 있나요?

Pharmacist: 치실은 4번 통로 중간 선반 위에 있고, 챕스틱은 3번 통로 맨 위의 선반 위에 있습니다.
Mr. Smith: 고맙습니다.

Pharmacist: 더 필요한 것이 있습니까?
Mr. Smith: 아닙니다.

Pharmacist: 다 합해서 $20.50입니다.
Mr. Smith: 지난번 약보다 가격이 저렴하군요.

Pharmacist: 음, 고객님이 처방 받은 약은 오리지널 약입니다. 오리지널 약은 상당히 비쌉니다. 그래서 고객님이 의사에게 카피약으로 처방해달라고 요청하셔서 이번에 가격이 더 저렴합니다. 아시다시피 카피약은 오리지널 약 가격의 반액이기 때문입니다.
Mr. Smith: 알겠습니다.

Pharmacist: 여기 약이 있습니다. 좋은 하루 되세요.
Mr. Smith: 약사님도요. 감사합니다.

2. 처방전
RX가 뜻하는 것은?

일부 사람들은 RX를 처방전이라고 생각합니다.
어떤 면에서는 맞습니다.
그러나, RX는 라틴어로 "조리법"이란 뜻입니다.

그림이 뜻하는 것은?

로리와 함께하는 미국문화 엿보기

"제가 환자분의 담당 의사 선생님의 필체를 이해하는데 고생했습니다. 하지만 드디어 제 생각에 처방전을 이해한 것 같습니다. 그렇지만, 만일 환자분이 주체할 수 없이 침을 질질 흘린다던가 10일 안에 체중이 약 9킬로그램 이상 증가한다면, 이 약을 즉시 중단하세요"

2. 처방전
처방전에 적혀있는 내용은?

1. 환자의 이름과 개인 정보 (나이, 주소, 생년월일)
2. *오늘 날짜*
3. 약 이름
4. 약 성분 함량
5. 한 번에 복용하는 양:

한 번에 복용하는 (알약, 주사, 기타 등등) 약의 1, 2, 3 또는 4번의 횟수를 "i, ii, iii 또는 iv" 로 표기합니다. 그리고 "sig"라는 용어가 복용할 횟수 앞에 빈번히 표기됩니다. ("sig"는 라틴어의 *signetur*의 약자로, "표기하시오"라는 뜻입니다.)

6. 약이 투여되는 (경구 또는 다른 방법) 경로를 의미합니다.

   복용방법:

   - **po** — 경구복용
   - **pr** — 좌약
   - **sl** — 설하제
   - **IV** — 정맥주사

- **IM** — 근육주사
- **SC** — 피하주사 (예를 들면 인슐린주사)
- **ID** — 피내주사 (예를 들면 튜베르쿨린 반응검사, 각종 약물의 앨러지 테스트(AST)에 이용)

7. 하루의 어느 시간, 공복 또는 음식과 함께 복용하는지 등 약의 복용 빈도와 방법에 관한 상세한 설명.

복용빈도:

- **qd** —하루에 한 번
- **bid** —하루에 두 번
- **tid** —하루에 세 번
- **qid** —하루에 네 번
- **q4h** —4시간 마다
- **qh** — 매 시간마다

예를 들어 약이 밤, 식전 또는 식후 등 특별한 방법으로 복용된다면 아래의 명칭이 빈도의 명칭 다음에 명시됩니다.

- **pc** —식 후
- **ac** —식 전
- **qhs** —잠자리에 들 때
- **prn** —필요 시

복약지시에 관한 추가 약자표기

tab: 알약

cap: 캡슐

pil: 작고 동그란 알약

syr: 시럽

gtt: 점액

ung: 연고

cr: 바르는 크림

od: 오른쪽 눈

os: 왼쪽 눈

tsp: 찻숟가락

tbsp: 숟가락

8. 한 번에 처방되는 약의 총 량 (예를 들면, 한 달치 또는 그 이상의 분량)

9. 다시 의사에게서 처방전을 받지 않고 같은 약을 재조제 받을 수 있는 횟수

재처방 받을 수 있는 횟수입니다. 예를 들면, "3RF"는 3회 재조제를 받을 수 있습니다.

10. 마약 단속반 번호

모든 처방전은 아니지만 일부 처방전은 의사의 마약 단속반 번호를 비롯한 추가 정보를 기재해야만 합니다. 예를 들면, 마약성 진통제와 같은 규제 성분이 들어 있는 약은 마약 단속반의 합당한 번호가 요구됩니다.

11. 의사의 서명

2. 처방전

연습문제: 아래의 빈칸에 알맞은 약자 (Abbreviation)를 적어 넣으세요.

Abbreviation	Meaning	Latin Term
ac	before meals	ante cibum
pc	after meals	post cibum
tab	tablet	tabella
cap	capsule	capsula
gtt	drop	gutta
hs	at bedtime	quaque hora somni
od	right eye	oculus dexter
os	left eye	oculus sinister
po	by mouth	per os
pil	pill	pilula
prn	as needed	pro re nata
q2h	every 2 hours	quaque 2 hora
qd	One/once a day	quaque die
qh	every hour	quaque hora
qid	4 times a day	quater in die
bid	twice a day	bis in die
tid	3 times a day	ter in die

2. 처방전
연습문제 처방전을 보고 아래의 질문(1-10)에 답하세요.
정답

1. What are the patient's name, address, and date of birth/age?

Patient's name: John Doe

Patient's address: Small Town, USA

Patient's date of birth/age: 53

2. What's the date today?

01/19 /2004

3. What's the name of the medication?

Ibuprofen

4. What's the dosage of the medication?

600 mg

5. How many doses should the medicine be taken at once?

1

6. By what route (oral or otherwise) should the medicine be administered?

By mouth/Orally

7. How often should the medicine be taken?

4 times a day

Also, are there any other details about how to take it, such as time of day, or with or without food?

After meal/(After meal & as needed)

If the medication is to be taken in a particular way — for example, at night, before food, or after food, then please describe it?

As needed/(After meal & as needed)

8. How many should the medicine be dispensed at once (e.g., one month supply or more)?

120

9. How many times can a patient get the prescription filled without getting his/her prescription issued again?

3 times

10. If patient's prescription contains narcotic substances, please write down the DEA number.

1234

2. 처방전
독해구문: 처방 받은 약병의 라벨 읽는 방법

지역 약국

약국 이름과 주소

(800) 555-5555

약국 전화번호

의사 존스 C.

의사선생님 성함

번호 0060023-08291

약의 재처방을 위해 약국에서 사용하는 약의 고유번호

2009 년 6 월 23 일

처방전 약을 받은 날짜

제인 스미스

이 약을 조제 받은 환자

처방 받은 약을 다 복용 할 때까지 10 일 동안 캡슐 한 개씩 하루에 세 번 경구 복용

얼마나 자주 그리고 언제 복용하는지에 관한 지시 사항

캡슐당 500 밀리그램 함량의 아막시실린

약의 이름과 함량

의사의 처방전 없이 약을 재조제 받을 수 있는 횟수

정해진 일자 전에 의사의 처방전 없이 약을 처방 받을 수 있는 횟수

2012 년 6 월 23 일 이전까지 사용

이 날짜가 지나면 약을 사용하지 마세요.

2. 처방전
약 처방받기

진료실에서

Dr. Mason: 스미스 선생님, 두 가지 약을 처방해 드리겠습니다. 한국으로 이 주 동안 출장을 가시기에 2주일 분량의 약을 처방했습니다.
Mr. Smith: 정말 감사합니다.

Dr. Mason: 처방한 약에 관해 설명을 드리겠습니다.
첫 번째 약은 소염제입니다.
이 약은 고관절의 염증을 완화할 것입니다.
하루에 알약 한 알씩 충분한 양의 물과 필요할 때마다 복용하세요.
Mr. Smith: 알겠습니다. 이 약이 통증도 완화시킵니까?

Dr. Mason: 예, 그렇습니다.
Mr. Smith: 정말 다행이군요.

Dr. Mason: 두 번째 약은 이뇨제입니다. 혈압이 아직도 높아요. 그래서 고혈압을 치료하기 위해 이뇨제를 처방했습니다. 하루에 한 알씩 복용하세요. 이해가 되셨습니까?
Mr. Smith: 예. 감사합니다.

Dr. Mason: 처방전은 밖에서 간호사 선생님한테 받아가세요.
다른 질문사항이 있나요?
Patient: 없습니다. 정말 감사합니다.

Dr. Mason: 천만에요. 출장 잘 다녀오세요.

3. 복약지시에 관한 주의사항
복약지시에 광한 주의사항 관련 주요구문

1. 이 약을 복용하시는 동안에 술 또는 담배를 피하세요.

2. 이 약을 다른 약과 함께 복용하지 마세요.

3. 잊지 말고 약을 복용하세요.

4. 항생제를 복용할 때 유제품을 피하세요. (제한해야 할 음식)

5. 공복에 약을 복용하지 마세요.

6. 처방 받은 약을 끝까지 다 복용하세요.

7. 차도가 있다고 복약을 중단하지 마세요. 치료를 끝까지 하지 않으면 재발하실 수 있습니다.

8. 가급적이면 매일 같은 시간에 약을 복용하세요.

9. 골다공증 약을 복용한 후 30분 동안은 눕지 마세요. 이와 같은 이유로, 잠자리에 들기 바로 전에 이 약을 복용하지 마세요.

10. 속 쓰림을 줄이기 위해 음식과 함께 복용하세요.

4. 약을 복용하는 방법
대화

식사 전 30분 복용

Jason: 당신은 얼마나 자주 약을 복용해야 하나요?
Jane: 약사 선생님이 식사하기 30분 전에 알약을 두 개씩 복용하라고 했어요.

식사 후 30분 복용

Patient: 항생제를 복용하기에 가장 좋은 시간이 언제인가요?
Pharmacist: 음, 항생제 복용에 가장 좋은 시간은 매 식사 후 30분 뒤입니다. 약병에 주의사항들이 적혀 있습니다. 위벽을 상하게 할 수 있으니 항생제를 공복에 복용하지 말도록 여기 적혀 있으므로, 식후 30분 뒤에 복용하세요.

식사와 함께/식사 후 즉시 복용

Max: 저녁준비 다 되었어요. 린다, 내 약을 가져다 줄래요?
Linda: 물론이죠. 그런데 당신은 약을 식사와 함께 복용하나요?

Max: 그래요. 의사선생님이 음식과 함께 복용하라고 해서, 매일 식사시간에 복용해야 해요.

취침 전에 복용

Herb doctor: 어디가 아프신가요?

Patient: 약 한달 동안 숙면을 취할 수가 없습니다. 하지만, 수면제를 처방받거나, 처방전 없이 구할 수 있는 수면제를 복용하고 싶지 않습니다. 수면제가 부작용이 있고 습관성이 될 수 있다는 사실이 염려됩니다.
더 나은 수면제를 추천해 주실 수 있습니까?

Herb doctor: 음, 그러면 내츄럴(생약성분) 수면제를 추천해 드리겠습니다. 내츄럴(생약성분) 수면제는 거의 부작용이 없고 습관성이 되지 않습니다. 복용해 보시겠습니까?

Patient: 예. 복용해 보겠습니다.

필요시 복용

Patient: 약 일주일 동안 마른기침과 인후염으로 고생하고 있습니다. 잘 듣는 목 캔디나 목 스프레이를 추천해 주시겠습니까?

Pharmacist: 물론이죠. 나는 이 목 캔디를 추천합니다. 이것은 인후염을 진정시키고, 마른 기침을 제거해줄 것입니다. 증상을 완화하기 위해 필요할 때마다 이 목 캔디를 드세요. 하지만, 기침이 계속 지속되고 차도가 있는 대신 더 악화되면 진료를 받으세요.

Patient: 알겠습니다. 감사합니다.

Pharmacist: 천만에요.

4. 약을 복용하는 방법
올바른 항생제 복용법

항생제를 처방 받았습니다.
만일 항생제를 오용하면, 염증을 치유하기가 더 어렵습니다.
아래의 중요한 설명들을 읽으세요.

항생제를 올바른 방법으로 복용하세요.

의료진들이 설명한대로 항생제를 복용하세요.

항생제 복용하는 것을 거르지 마세요.

다른 사람과 함께 복용하지 마세요.

나중에 사용하기 위해 남겨놓지 마세요.

상태가 호전되더라도 처방 받은 항생제를 다 드세요.

5. 약국에서 자주하는 질문
주요구문

Patient: 제가 이 약을 복용하기 전에 주의해야 할 사항이 있나요?

Pharmacist: 예. 이 약을 공복에 복용하지 마세요.

Patient: 이 약을 복용 중에 금주해야 하나요?

Pharmacist: 예. 이 약을 복용 중에는 금주하셔야 합니다.

Patient: 약 복용법을 알려주시겠습니까?

Pharmacist: 처방 받은 약병에 적혀 있습니다. 복약지시대로 드시면 됩니다.

Patient: 약 복용하는 것을 어떻게 기억할 수 있을까요?

Pharmacist: 일주일 분량의 약을 요일 별로 나누어 담는 용기를 약국에서 구입하세요. 약을 잊지 않고 복용하시는데 도움이 되실 것입니다.

Patient: 이 연고를 어떻게 바르나요?

Pharmacist: 매일 아침 얇게 연고를 바르시고 거즈를 붙이세요.

Patient: 제 약을 냉장고에 보관해야 하나요?

Pharmacist: 실내온도로 보관하시고 지나친 열기 및 습기가 있는 곳은 피하세요(화장실에 보관하지 마세요). 또한 약은 원래의 약병에 밀폐시켜서 보관하시고, 어린이들의 손에 닿지 않는 곳에 보관 하세요. 약은 의사 또는 약사의 지시에 따라 보관하세요.

Patient: 만일 차도가 있으면 복용을 중단해도 되나요?

Pharmacist: 의사선생님의 승인 없이는 갑자기 중단하지 마세요.

다 드실 때까지 규칙적으로 복용하세요.

Patient: 이 약을 복용한 후 운전을 해도 되나요?

Pharmacist: 이 약을 복용한 후 졸릴 수 있으므로 운전은 하지 않는 것이 최선입니다.

Patient: 약을 어떻게 처방 받지요?

Pharmacist: 처방전을 약국에 가져오시고 약을 받으시면 됩니다.

Patient: 목 캔디와 소독약 팔아요?

Pharmacist: 예. 팝니다.

6. 비처방전 약
독해구문

약 효과 성분(각각의 알약) **용도**

Chlorpheniramine maleate 2 mg .... 항히스타민제

효능. 효과 꽃가루 앨러지 또는 상기도 호흡기 앨러지 증상의 일시적인 증상의 완화:

- 재채기
- 콧물
- 가렵고 눈물이 나는 눈
- 간질거리는 목

주의사항

만일 아래와 같은 증상이 있다면 사용전(복용전) 의사와 상의 하세요

- 녹내장
- 기관지 확장증 또는 만성기관지염과 같은 호흡기 질환
- 전립선 비대로 인한 배뇨 장애

만일 신경안정제 또는 진정제를 복용 중이라면 이 약을 복용하기 전에 의사 또는 약사와 상의하세요.

이 약을 복용하실 때

- 졸릴 수 있습니다.
- 술을 삼가하세요.
- 술, 진정제, 신경안정제는 졸리움을 유발할 수 있습니다.
- 운전을 하거나 기계를 작동할 때 주의하세요.
- 특히 어린아이들에게서 흥분 상태가 일어날 수 있습니다.

만일 임신 중이거나 또는 모유 수유 중일 경우, 약을 복용하기 전에 의료진과 상의 하세요.

아이들의 손에 닿지 않는 곳에 보관 하세요.

과다 복용을 한 경우, 즉시 의료진에 도움을 요청하던가 독극물관리센터에 연락하세요.

복약지시

12세 이상-성인	4시간에서 6시간 마다 2정을 복용하세요; 24시간 내에 12정 이상은 복용하지 마세요.
6세-12세 미만	4시간에서 6시간 마다 1정을 복용하세요; 24시간 내에 6정 이상은 복용하지 마세요.
6세 미만의 소아	의사와 상의 하세요.

기타정보 섭씨20-25도(실온)에서 보관하세요. (화씨로는 68-77도입니다.)

- 지나치게 습기가 많은 곳은 피하세요.

비활성 성분 D&C 노란색 번호 10번인 식용 염료, 락토스, 스테아린산 마그네슘(식품첨가물), 미세결정 셀룰로스(첨가제), 호화(알파)전분.

6. 비처방전 약 대화구문

비처방전 코막힘 약

Pharmacist: 무엇을 도와드릴까요?

Customer: 2~3일 동안 코가 꽉 막혀서 고생하고 있어요.

코 막힌데 좋은 약을 추천해 주시겠습니까?

Pharmacist: 이 코 힘 약을 추천해 드리겠습니다. 매우 효과적입니다.

Customer: 좋아요. 몇 알씩 복용해야 하나요?

Pharmacist: 하루에 세 알씩 드세요.

Customer: 음, 제가 건망증이 심해요. 그래서 만일에 약 복용하는 것을 잊으면 어떻게 하나요?

Pharmacist: 음. 만일 복용량을 한번 걸렀고, 한 시간 안에 기억한다면, 곧바로 드세요.

Customer: 알겠습니다. 하지만 한참 후에 기억한다면, 복용을 하지 못한 약을 함께 두 배로 복용해야 하나요?

Pharmacist: 복용하지 못한 약은 거르시고 다시 복용 일정을 따라주세요. 그리고 결코 약을 두 배로 복용하지 마세요. 이해 되십니까?

Customer: 예. 그런데 부작용이 있나요?

Pharmacist: 음, 일부 환자들이 어지러움과 메스꺼움을 호소했습니다. 또한, 이 약은 졸음을 유발하므로, 복용 후 운전하지 마세요.

Customer: 운전하지 않겠습니다.

Pharmacist: 다른 질문사항이 있습니까?

Customer: 없습니다. 정말 감사합니다.

Pharmacist: 천만에요. 하지만 증상이 더 악화된다면, 의사 선생님에게 진찰을 받으셔야 합니다.